Reading the Psychosomatic in Medical and Popular Culture

Pain. Chronic digestive symptoms. Poor sleep. Neuropathy. Sensory disturbances. Fatigue. Panic. Constant illness and discomfort. Frequent difficulty coping with work, school, relationships.

Despite the common experience of being told that it's all in their heads, that they're *just making themselves sick*, individuals with these symptoms are experiencing a very real, sometimes debilitating, illness phenomenon. But what is it? Physical or mental illness? Political or social identity? Cultural, narrative, or discursive construction? When something goes awry at the intersection of mind and body – the psychosomatic – what is happening?

Widely recognized, yet difficult to classify, diagnose, treat, and explain, psychosomatic disorders are heavily stigmatized, and the associated syndromes have become the site of controversy and antipathy in the provider–patient relationship. In popular culture, terms such as medically unexplained symptoms, hysteria, neurasthenia, hypochondria, functional illness, and malingering are misunderstood, unknown, or rejected outright. Meanwhile, perspectives from cultural and textual studies focus on the psychosomatic as a metaphor in art, literature, and popular media, where disruptions of the body and mind are regularly made to stand in for individual alienation and cultural malaise. Bringing together multiple perspectives, this challenging volume tackles causes, and innovative, humanistic solutions, to conflicts in the provider–patient relationship; uses the psychosomatic as a lens for theorizing the self in culture; and examines the metaphorical potential of the psychosomatic in fictional narrative.

Providing a unique assemblage of interdisciplinary, international approaches to understanding the problem of the psychosomatic in both expert and lay discourses, this pioneering edited collection is aimed at students and researchers of health, popular culture, and the health care humanities.

Carol-Ann Farkas is Associate Professor of English in the School of Arts and Sciences at Massachusetts College of Pharmacy and Health Sciences (MCPHS), Boston, USA.

Routledge Advances in the Medical Humanities

https://www.routledge.com/Routledge-Advances-in-Disability-Studies/book-series/RADS

New titles

Dementia and Literature
Cross-disciplinary Perspectives
Edited by Tess Maginess

Reading the Psychosomatic in Medical and Popular Culture
Something. Nothing. Everything
Edited by Carol-Ann Farkas

Medicine, Health and the Arts
Approaches to the Medical Humanities
Edited by Victoria Bates, Alan Bleakley and Sam Goodman

Suffering Narratives of Older Adults
A Phenomenological Approach to Serious illness, Chronic Pain, Recovery and Maternal Care
Mary Beth Morrissey

Medical Humanities and Medical Education
How the Medical Humanities Can Shape Better Doctors
Alan Bleakley

Learning Disability and Inclusion Phobia
Past, Present and Future
C. F. Goodey

Collaborative Arts-based Research for Social Justice
Victoria Foster

Forthcoming titles

The Experience of Institutionalisation
Social Exclusion, Stigma and Loss of Identity
Jane Hubert

Reading the Psychosomatic in Medical and Popular Culture

Something. Nothing. Everything

Edited by Carol-Ann Farkas

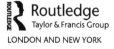

Routledge
Taylor & Francis Group

LONDON AND NEW YORK

First published 2018
by Routledge
2 Park Square, Milton Park, Abingdon, Oxon OX14 4RN

and by Routledge
605 Third Avenue, New York, NY 10017

First issued in paperback 2021

Routledge is an imprint of the Taylor & Francis Group, an informa business

Publisher's Note
The publisher has gone to great lengths to ensure the quality of this reprint but points out that some imperfections in the original copies may be apparent.

British Library Cataloguing-in-Publication Data
A catalogue record for this book is available from the British Library

Library of Congress Cataloging-in-Publication Data
Names: Farkas, Carol-Ann, editor.
Title: Reading the psychosomatic in medical and popular culture : something. nothing. everything / edited by Carol-Ann Farkas.
Description: Milton Park, Abingdon, Oxon : Routledge, 2018. | Includes bibliographical references and index.
Identifiers: LCCN 2017012360 | ISBN 9781138699977 (hbk) | ISBN 9781315515694 (ebk)
Subjects: LCSH: Medicine, Psychosomatic. | Physician and patient.
Classification: LCC RC49 .R43 2018 | DDC 616.08—dc23
LC record available at https://lccn.loc.gov/2017012360

ISBN 13: 978-0-367-34150-3 (pbk)
ISBN 13: 978-1-138-69997-7 (hbk)
ISBN 13: 978-1-315-51569-4 (ebk)

DOI: 10.4324/9781315515694

Typeset in Times New Roman
by Apex CoVantage, LLC

Contents

vi   *Contents*

Editor

Carol-Ann Farkas is Associate Professor of English in the School of Arts and Sciences at Massachusetts College of Pharmacy and Health Sciences (MCPHS) where she directs and teaches in the first-year English program, and teaches elective and directed study courses in nineteenth-century fiction and narrative and medicine. As a scholar with a background in Victorian, cultural, and composition studies, she currently specializes in the interdisciplinary study of medicine and wellness in popular culture. Previous publications have focused on the gendered representation of physical competence in popular fitness magazines ("Bodies at rest, bodies in motion: Women's fitness and physical competence," in *Genders Online*), the wellness "education" constructed by fitness magazines ("'Tons of useful stuff': Defining wellness in popular magazines," in *Studies in Popular Culture*), the teaching of literature and medicine in a health sciences context ("Teaching madness and literature in a healthcare context: An enquiry into interdisciplinary education," in *Mental Health Review Journal*, co-authored with David Flood), and, most recently, the ways in which popular media contribute to the experience of psychosomatic illness ("Potentially harmful side-effects: Medically unexplained symptoms, somatization, and the failed illness narrative for viewers of mystery diagnosis," in *The Journal of Medical Humanities*, and "The blind men and the elephant: Mediating conflicting views of controversial diagnoses," in *Trespassing*). She is a past president of the Northeast Popular Culture Studies Association and is currently Chair of the Health, Disease, and Wellness Area for the Popular Culture Association in the USA; she is also part of the Center for Health Care Humanities at MCPHS University, a group which fosters the interdisciplinary scholarship and teaching of the medical humanities.

Contributors

Seamus L. Barker has worked as a physiotherapist, mainly in Pain Clinics in Australia, for over ten years. Concurrently, he completed a BA (Hons) in English and Social Theory at the University of Melbourne (Australia), and an MPhil in English at the University of Cambridge (UK). Currently he is a PhD candidate at the University of Sydney, supervised by Professor Chris Jordens (bioethics) and Professor John Frow (English). He is also supervised by Professor G. Lorimer Moseley. Barker's PhD investigates what is at stake in the discrepancies between different accounts of pain coming from scientific and medical discourses, and from personal narratives. He and Professor Moseley are interested in understanding and overcoming barriers to the way in which pain is understood and successfully managed at all levels of society.

Hilde Bondevik is an Associate Professor at the Department of Health Sciences, the Medical Faculty, The University of Oslo. Her background is the history of ideas and gender studies. Her main research interests relate to cultural aspects of health and illness, medical history, gender perspectives on health and illness, literature and medicine, and the philosophy of science. She has published several books, including one about the hysteria diagnosis and its history in Norway. She has also published several papers in international journals, including the recent articles "Medical constructions of long-term exhaustion – past and present," *Sociology of Health and Illness* (with Olaug S. Lian, 2015), and "Absent organs – Present selves: Exploring embodiment and gender identity in young Norwegian women's accounts of hysterectomy," *International Journal of Qualitative Studies on Health and Well-being* (with Kari Nyheim Solbrække, 2015).

Paola Chesi has worked as a researcher at Fondazione ISTUD – Health Care Area since 2010. She graduated in Natural Science from the University of Torino and has been working in the field of research. She is an expert in the analysis of patient care and social organization, focusing in particular on the areas of narrative medicine and medical humanities. She is involved in several national and international projects, and coordinates training courses on narrative medicine.

Claire Hooker is Senior Lecturer and Coordinator of Health Humanities at the Centre for Values, Ethics and Law, University of Sydney, and a foundation member of the Sydney Arts and Health Collective. Her research interests include arts and health; health risk issue management; building supportive, high-quality work environments in health care, and building empathy in health care.

Olaug S. Lian is a Professor in Medical Sociology at the Department of Community Medicine, University of Tromsø – The Arctic University of Norway, where she currently leads the research group Medical Humanities. She also works part-time as a Research Advisor at the University Hospital of Northern Norway. Her research interests relate to cultural aspects of health and illness, health services, and the role of health professionals. She has published three books and several papers in high-impact international journals, most notably in *Qualitative Health Research:* "'I do not really belong out there any more.' Sense of being and belonging among people with medically unexplained long-term fatigue" (with Geir Lorem, 2016); *Journal of Medical Humanities:* "Generating a social movement online community through an online discourse: The case of myalgic encephalomyelitis (with Jan Grue, 2016), and *Sociology of Health and Illness:* "Medical constructions of long-term exhaustion – past and present" (with Hilde Bondevik, 2015).

Maria Giulia Marini is an epidemiologist and counselor with a classic humanistic background, and a background in scientific academic studies, chemistry, and pharmacology. She began her career in medical research before moving to health care organization, with an academic specialization in epidemiology. She is now a researcher and counselor at Fondazione ISTUD, applying principles of humanistic management to health care. She is currently on the board of the Italian Society of Narrative Medicine, is a tenured Professor of Narrative Medicine at Hunimed, Milan, and a referee for WHO for "Narrative Method in Public Health."

G. Lorimer Moseley is Professor of Clinical Neurosciences and Chair of Physiotherapy of the University of South Australia. He is Chair of PainAdelaide Stakeholders' Consortium, and leads the Body in Mind Research Group, based at University of South Australia and at Neuroscience Australia, Sydney. He researches the role of the brain and mind in chronic pain, and has written several books, published 225 papers, and regularly presents and teaches around the world. Together with Seamus Barker, he recently wrote "The difficult problem: Chronic pain and the politics of care" for *Australian Quarterly, 87*(3), 2016, 8–17.

Daniele De Nardo is a medical doctor. During the course of the ISTUD study on fibromyalgia he worked at the Department of Medical, Surgical and Health Sciences of the University of Trieste; currently he works at the Department of Internal Medicine of Riuniti Hospital of Trieste, Italy.

Jessica Parr is a PhD candidate at the University of New South Wales in Sydney, Australia. Her thesis will consider the medical and popular responses to obesity in postwar America and recent publications, based on her doctoral research, have appeared in *Social History of Medicine* (2014) and *Critical Perspectives on Addiction* (2012).

Camelia Raghinaru holds a PhD in English from the University of Florida, and currently works as an Assistant Professor of English at Concordia University, Irvine. Her research interests focus on utopian studies, modernism, and popular culture. Her articles on Conrad, Lawrence, Joyce, Woolf, and Bréton have been published in various academic journals (*Studies in the Novel, [sic], Forum*, etc.) and edited collections (*Great War Modernism* and *Critical Approaches to Joseph Conrad*). Currently she is working on two essays dealing with the shift from Victorianism to modernism in Joseph Conrad and popular modernisms in recent TV shows.

Luigi Reale is Project Coordinator for the Health Research Foundation ISTUD. He has a Masters in Healthcare Management from SDA Bocconi in Milan. He has worked on implementing a system of management control and functional organization to be applied in university hospitals. His research projects have centered on training and development relating to the reorganization of diagnostic and therapeutic care, and economic evaluations according to a socio-medical approach to integrated governance in health. His current research interests are in the complex world of disabilities and neurodegenerative diseases and home care settings.

Catherine Robson is a post-doctoral researcher with a background in sociology, health science, and medical social work. She is particularly interested in the study of clinical interactions involving people with functional neurological symptoms, and exploring the perspectives of people who live with these conditions and those who help treat and care for them. Her PhD (University of York, UK) explored diagnostic differences in how people with epilepsy and people with psychogenic non-epileptic seizures describe their experiences in film recordings of 70 outpatient neurology consultations. More recently, she critically examined how neurologists name and explain the cause of medically unexplained seizures to patients (with Olaug. S. Lian, 2016); *Forum: Qualitative Social Research:* "Are you saying she's mentally ill then?"). She is currently involved in two projects related to studying the experience of patients with medically unexplained symptoms.

Caryn Kseniya Rubanovich is a graduate of the M.S. Narrative Medicine Program at Columbia University in the City of New York, where she studied clinician–patient relationships and patient care. She is currently a research study coordinator at the Center for Behavioral Intervention Technologies at Northwestern University where she works with an interdisciplinary team, bridging gaps in mental health care with innovative technologies. She aims to apply for doctoral programs in clinical psychology, to investigate mental health and well-being among physicians and medical students.

Amba J. Sepie has an academic and teaching background in anthropology, religious studies, and sociology, and a "real-world" background in holistic and traditional medicines. She is currently completing her doctorate in the field of cultural geography at the University of Canterbury in Christchurch, New Zealand. Her research and publications center on decolonization in the intersecting areas of medicine and education, with a focus on social justice outcomes through the direct engagement with other ways of knowing and being. Her most recent publications on these topics include a paper on "Heretical anthropology" in *Symbolism: An International Annual of Critical Aesthetics, 16*, 295–313, a chapter in *Damned Facts: Fortean Essays on Religion, Folklore and the Paranormal*, edited by Jack Hunter, and "Conversing with some chickadees: Cautious acts of ontological translation," *Literature and Medicine, 32*(2), 2014, 277–298.

Louise Stone is a general practitioner in Canberra, Australia and a Senior Lecturer at the Australian National University Academic Unit of General Practice. She has extensive clinical experience managing patients with complex mental illness and medically unexplained symptoms in primary care. She is a medical educator with expertise in online learning, and has delivered courses and workshops in mental illness, especially to rural and remote doctors, for over 20 years. She completed her PhD in 2014, exploring the way in which novice and experienced GPs assess and manage patients with medically unexplained illness.

Maria Tutorskaya is Head of the Methodical Cabinet at the Center for the Development of the Russian History of Medicine Museums at Moscow State University of Medicine and Dentistry (MSUMD). She graduated from the MSU, where she specialized in history and anthropology. Thereafter she gained specialist degree in Nursing and worked as a History of Medicine lecturer in the First MSUMD for almost ten years. Her research and pedagogical interests include medical humanities, in particular literature and medicine and medical anthropology. Together with her colleague Elena Berger, she is an editor of three anthologies for medical students: a collection of medical texts; a collection of fiction narratives describing the doctor's path from medical school to the end of the professional career; and a collection of essays on dentistry in popular literature. She was awarded a Fulbright Faculty Development Program grant in 2015. She developed a course description, syllabus, and outline for a course in literature and medicine under the supervision of Dr. Carol-Ann Farkas at MCPHS University. Currently she is implementing newly gained knowledge and experience at the MSUMD in Moscow.

Hannah Tweed is Co-Director of the Scottish Universities International Summer School, based at the University of Edinburgh. She was awarded her PhD from the University of Glasgow in 2015, where she then worked as a Teaching Fellow in English literature, and as a researcher for the Medical Humanities Research Centre. Her thesis focused on representations of autism in contemporary literature and film, drawing upon disability studies and work from within the medical humanities. In addition to a monograph based on her PhD thesis, she is working on a project on contagion in contemporary literature. She is the co-founder of the Disability Studies Network UK, and runs the website for the Glasgow Medical Humanities Research Centre. She reviews regularly for *Disability Studies Quarterly, H-Disability, The Year's Work in English Studies,* and *The Journal of Literary and Cultural Disability Studies.*

Acknowledgments

Reading the Psychosomatic in Medical and Popular Culture: Something. Nothing. Everything exists thanks to the innovative, erudite, and diligent work of our international group of contributors from the USA, Australia, New Zealand, Norway, Italy, UK, and Russia: endless thanks to Caryn, Maria Giulia, Paola, Luigi, Daniele, Claire, Louise, Amba, Seamus, Masha, Jessica, Hilde, Olaug, Catherina, Camelia, and Hannah. We are all grateful for the support of our editorial team at Routledge, who have made this anthology a reality.

I am deeply appreciative of all of the people who have encouraged me professionally and personally in this work. I extend thanks to my institution, MCPHS University, for its ongoing support of this important research, in particular the Center for Health Care Humanities, founded by David Tanner to promote scholarship and teaching in this essential discipline. Jennifer Tebbe Grossman receives an extra-special thank-you for her mentorship and guidance throughout my career as a researcher. Finally, all the gratitude in the world goes to my family and friends for their encouragement, reassurance, support, and occasional hand-holding: thank you Ted, Ivy, Kate, and Peter.

Introduction

The psychosomatic as nothing, something, and everything

Carol-Ann Farkas

Everyone has had – or will have – psychosomatic illness at some point in their lives. Insofar as your body (soma) and mind (psyche) respond to the conditions of your life in ways which are unpredictable, and often undesirable, you have almost certainly had an illness experience which was medically unexplained, its etiology unknown or unrecognized, and – this is the important part – to which you and people in your life ascribed varied explanations, or from which you inferred potential meanings. You may be going about the business of your life, dealing with its challenges just fine, until you start to have odd aches and pains, an oddly vulnerable immune system, digestive trouble, fatigue, inflammation, poor sleep, neuropathy, or sensory disturbance, which, singly or in combination, may be naggingly irritating or fully debilitating, interfering with work, school, relationships, *everything.* And when the symptoms neither go away nor yield to explanation or diagnosis, someone (a doctor, a friend, a partner) may suggest that perhaps it's *nothing,* that you're just under too much stress, that you're a hypochondriac, that you're making yourself sick, that these symptoms are simply "all in your head" – that your symptoms must mean *something* else, about your health, your identity, even your place in the world.

The psychosomatic, when taken at its simplest and most denotative, should not be as problematic as it is. After all, what *isn't* psychosomatic? When does affective, cognitive, or psychological distress *not* affect the body? When does the body's condition – as we perceive it, think about it, react to it, and respond to others' reactions – not affect the mind? And yet to suggest that something is psychosomatic is to invoke stigmatizing connotations of discomfort, resistance, and maddening uncertainty. What is happening? When the psychosomatic intrudes, when something goes inexplicably awry at the intersection of mind and body, what is it? Physical or mental illness? Political or social identity? Cultural, narrative, and/or discursive construction? What does the "psychosomatic" mean as a biopsychosocial disorder? As a cultural phenomenon? As a metaphor?

The central problem of the "psychosomatic" is that we all have it, diagnose it, use it, but none of us – laypeople, and experts in medicine, psychology, the social sciences, and cultural and textual studies – are talking about the same thing, in the same place, for the same purposes. Specialists in medicine, psychology, and sociology engage in ongoing debate (with one another, rarely with patients themselves) about how to classify, diagnose, treat, and explain disorders which affect body and mind, and which play a role in as many as 50 percent of clinical visits to healthcare providers. Yet "psychosomatic" illness is heavily stigmatized, and the associated syndromes have become the site of controversy and antipathy in the provider–patient relationship. In popular culture, terms such as medically unexplained symptoms, hysteria, neurasthenia, hypochondria, psychogenic illness, somatic symptoms, functional illness, and malingering are largely unknown, misunderstood, or rejected outright. At the same time, we seek names, definitions, explanations for the inexplicable symptoms which bedevil us; we educate ourselves about unexplained and controversial symptoms through varied self-help and wellness-themed media; we advocate for and with one another through social media; we consume and produce narratives about the inextricability of the body and mind in fiction, television, and film – and rarely does the term "psychosomatic" actually appear. Meanwhile, scholars focus on the "psychosomatic" vis-à-vis its figurative potential as a metaphor in art, literature, and popular media, where disruptions of the body and mind are regularly made to stand in for individual alienation and cultural malaise.

We can see that there has been abundant study and deployment of the "psychosomatic" in numerous disciplines and multiple discourses, and yet there has been little interdisciplinary inquiry which brings together competing, complementary perspectives. This anthology is an attempt to bridge some of the knowledge gaps which confuse communication across and between these different constituents – experts and laypeople; the sciences, social sciences, and humanities – fraught (at best), ineffectual to non-existent (at worst). The essays here are not intended to provide a clinical explanation of what the psychosomatic is, at least not in the sense of providing empirically-observable measures for etiology, diagnosis, or reliable therapy. The symptoms and syndromes which align with the psychosomatic remain disputed sites of authority and identity . . . and this collection will not resolve that contest. Indeed, these essays will likely complicate your understanding before they provide clarity. This is exactly what we believe makes this collection so valuable: rather than explain what the psychosomatic *is*, the authors assembled here all seek to understand what the psychosomatic *does*, what uses we put it to, and what work it does for us: medically, socially, and culturally. Rather than attempting to simplify, define, or disambiguate, the authors here wade right into the murky, unsettled waters of the psychosomatic to explore how a phenomenon that is so chaotic can be capable of so much suffering, upheaval, disorder – and meaning.

To what extent does our identity as "ill" or "well" depend on the relationship between our minds and our bodies? Pay attention to your *self* as you move through your life: can you easily draw a sharp distinction between your bodily experience, and the thoughts and feelings which come and go as motivation for and response to that experience? That you can ponder this question demonstrates Descartes' great insight: *cogito, ergo sum* (I think, therefore I am); that you take for granted that your self is a whole entity comprised of two disparate parts demonstrates the way in which Cartesian dualism has become enshrined not only in medical culture but also in the larger popular culture as a fundamental premise in our concept of health and illness. The biomedical model, predominant in both expert and popular cultures since the Enlightenment, leads us to assume that, in general, illness works, and signifies – mechanically, biochemically, socially, and ethically – very differently in the body than it does in the mind. The fundamental premise remains dualistic: we are made up of two parts which should, optimally, function cooperatively and complementarily, but which can, sub-optimally, become misaligned and dis-integrated, to work antagonistically against one another. Even now, in the early twenty-first century, as we undertake varied measures to improve wellness through integrative, mind–body practices, our unexamined assumption is that we must take charge of the more biddable part as a way of rehabilitating the other, recalcitrant part.

We apply this dualistic model unfairly, selectively, and inconsistently. How can we do otherwise, when the model is almost certainly – though we may not yet know why – wrong, or at least, overly simplistic and incomplete? As we begin to understand just how complicated the human organism is – from our experience of pain, to the ways in which the microbiome influences physiology, mood, and cognition through the brain–gut axis, to the relationship of musculoskeletal movement with the stress response (Dum *et al.*, 2016) – it becomes increasingly inaccurate to consider the mind and the body as though they are distinct and independently functioning entities. An insistence on dualism leaves no space at all for the role of social relationships and culture in the health of individuals. Far from being a dismissive, "waste-basket" diagnosis (Dimsdale, 2011, p. 55), the complexity of the psychosomatic makes it a potentially vital concept to include as we move towards a more biopsychosocial (Engel, 1977) understanding of wellness.

Yet (centuries-old) habits die hard. The biomedical model has been invaluable for advancing knowledge through empirical study. However, as we have privileged (perhaps necessarily) that which can be observed, quantified, and explained, we have marginalized that which is inexplicable, that which exceeds the sophistication of science and its practitioners. The desire for certainty renders ambiguity intolerable (Montgomery, 2006) – and nothing is more intolerable than an illness which has no distinct, discernible, unambiguous mechanism.

All the more exasperating is that the experience, the affliction of such medically unexplained ambiguity is so common. Medically unexplained symptoms (MUS) account for a significant proportion – between 15 and 50 percent – of visits to both primary care and specialists (Barsky *et al.*, 2005; Ring, 2005)[1]. The underlying problem might be something trivial; it might be something acute, violent, but ultimately transient; or it might be a constellation of chronic, pernicious symptoms, under the rubric of chronic fatigue syndrome (CFS), myalgic encephalopathy (ME), or fibromyalgia, all of which are highly contested diagnoses amongst experts and lay people. Those who have identified themselves as CFS or Fibromyalgia sufferers often understand their illness as purely physiological, and a multitude of studies concur; however, many researchers also agree that there is some psychogenic component: that is, that the patient's experience of bodily distress is caused, or exacerbated, by disordered cognitive and/or affective responses

(Barsky *et al.*, 2005; Ring *et al.*, 2005; Creed, 2012). Although "psychogenic" is meant to be a more neutral term than the more stigmatizing "psychosomatic" which, in North American culture in particular, has a long and uncomfortable association with "hysteria," I have argued elsewhere that "biopsychosocial" is a better descriptor for such conditions (Farkas, 2014).

Here is the basis of patient–provider conflict at its worst and most antagonistic. Providers, having passed through the formal and "hidden" curricula of medical education, and working within an under-resourced healthcare system, have incomplete knowledge, often acquired along with an abundance of stigmatizing beliefs about the medically unexplained, the intolerably ambiguous, or "psychosomatic" (Nettleton, 2006; Shattock *et al.*, 2013). Even the most sympathetic providers, when confronted with illness that is not, clinically, "disease," have no better strategies for countering patients' subjective beliefs, beyond offering interpretations which are no more empirically valid, but which carry the weight of expert experience, knowledge, and cultural capital. It is little wonder that patients are not more biddable when their "evidence" seems no more reliable than the physician's: "It is a difficult concept to grasp. It is an idea for which there is no proof and on which there is still no consensus . . . I believe in and accept the unconscious, uncontrollable nature of psychosomatic disability" (O'Sullivan, 2015, pp. 144–148).

Meanwhile, patients come to the clinical encounter with an intensely physical, "real" experience of symptoms, for which popular health discourses (from fictional television to the multifarious information of the internet) have provided accessible and plausible diagnoses. We laypeople, as well trained as the experts to trust the biomedical model, experience significant bewilderment and frustration when its practitioners cannot help us, when they are as baffled by our symptoms as we are. Particularly provoking is the feeling (often justified) that physicians are not taking their patients seriously – where, as Belling (2006) puts it, the patient's interpretive reading challenges the physician's "evidence-based" measures and practices, and is consequently met with a great deal of provider scepticism. The suspicion, or interpretation, that the patient's symptoms are all in her head, or even just not "clinically relevant", is maddening (Shapiro, 2011; Shattock *et al.*, 2013; Barker, 2011).

Thus "psychosomatic" becomes one of many terms coined over the centuries not just to describe and diagnose, but to assess. Inherent in the use of the term is a medico-moral judgment by one group or another, wherein psychosomatic patients are stigmatized as difficult: the symptoms which comprise their disorder seem suspiciously like an affront to order. These are the "heartsink" patients who are said to try the patience of the expert with their non-adherent (non-compliant) resistance to advice, and their inconsistent and chaotic narratives (Stone, 2014). Patients who have felt that their providers treat them dismissively, condescendingly, or judgmentally turn to one another through social media and use their shared "non-expert" space to reinforce their sense of grievance, antagonism, and mistrust of the experts as they pursue the authorization of their illness experience (Barker, 2008). The psychosomatic categorization, in turn, provokes the behavior it is meant to constrain: recalcitrant patients, displaced from the validation of the sick role, turn against medical authority and towards one another for support and knowledge. Using a variety of resources, shared directly and indirectly through the internet, not only do patients educate themselves about symptoms and treatments, but they reinforce their identification with both disorder and political cause (Barker, 2008, 2011).

The combination of frustration, antagonism, distress, resistance, stigmatization, and uncertainty which characterize the psychosomatic as a clinical problem are – oh-so-perversely – what give it signifying force as an element in narrative. Indeed, the ambiguity of the psychosomatic is a powerful driver of "effort after meaning"; the need to impose coherence where there is none (Bartlett, 1932). We create stories about how our minds and bodies can, should, will, or won't cooperate; but the psychosomatic story defies our desire for stable characters, and a linear, resolved (acute, never chronic) plot which follows the "mythological" patterns of journeys and battles (Hawkins, 1999). Far from the ideal narrative of "restitution," as long as symptoms remain unexplained, the narrative can be nothing but one of chaos, a failure (Frank, 1995; Hydén, 1997). In particular, we can read the unresolved/unresolvable conflicts inherent in the psychosomatic as *failures of relationships*, where the literal disconnect provides the material for the analogous, the figurative, the metaphorical: for mind versus body; individual versus family, society, culture. The psychosomatic-as-metaphor epitomizes what Mitchell and Snyder (2001) refer to as the prosthesis of narrative conflict – a symbol for that which is disabled or broken in the plot, in our lives, a wound which offers a site for response – potentially to heal, or more provocatively, to challenge, resisting the illusory, normative, disciplinary "healing" demanded of the contemporary neoliberal subject.

The authors in this collection represent very different disciplinary perspectives and methods – from sociology to textual studies to medicine – but they are assembled here out of a shared concern with the cultural work done by, and through, the discourses of the psychosomatic. While we cannot explain the mechanisms that generate symptoms in the mind and body, we can collectively examine the myriad ways in which literal pain and discomfort are produced by, and productive of, figurative discourses of illness. How do beliefs and assumptions about health and wholeness drive us to read the psychosomatic as a metaphor? How do the illness and brokenness of the psychosomatic, in turn, function metaphorically to illustrate all manner of other conflicts, other sites of what is *broken*, throughout our culture?

We start with the clinic, with Caryn Rubanovich's examination of the psychosomatic as an intractable conflict in the provider–patient relationship. She is concerned with the limitations of Western biomedicine as both an explanatory paradigm and a set of institutional practices, resulting in contested claims to knowledge, authority, and care. Providers and patients will not, because they cannot, agree on how to interpret the psychosomatic. By the time both parties meet in the consulting room, their beliefs about how mind and body interact have been shaped by the discourses of health which prevail in both medical education and within the larger culture. The psychosomatic defies attempts to manage or care.

Whatever the presumed underlying, *literal* pathology may be, the psychosomatic asserts itself as a manifestation of the *figurative* pathology which afflicts not just healthcare but all our systems of care. In response, Rubanovich sets the tone for this collection by offering a strategy with therapeutic potential: she provides a rationale for a model of applied medical humanities, where the practices of creating and interpreting texts, telling and reading stories, may be used to help providers and patients construct more compassionate narratives of healing.

In Chapter 2, Maria Giulia Marini, Daniele De Nardo, Paola Chesi, and Luigi Reale provide a model of these principles in direct clinical practice. Of the syndromes which have historically fallen under the heading of the psychosomatic, fibromyalgia is one of the more fraught, contested sites for provider–patient conflict – and debilitating distress for those individuals living with its symptoms. Observing this conflict, the group theorized that improved communication, nurtured through a structured sharing of narratives, might help. In their study, both patients and their doctor kept journals wherein they could each articulate their experience of being ill and receiving treatment for the illness. Both groups found that the practice of reflective writing, in and of itself, had a therapeutic effect. Using a framework of transactional analysis, Marini *et al.* map the progress of patients and physicians as they use narrative to negotiate the threats posed by illness to individual and social identity. These stories also afforded their physician valuable insight into their concerns, forcibly reminding him of their humanity in a way that helped heal the conflicts provoked by the contestation surrounding their diagnoses. The doctor in the study was able to see that although he and his patients might not easily agree on how to account for, and name, their symptoms, their sharing of narrative was a crucial step in putting their health right through their collective agreement that there was definitely *something* wrong.

But what happens, ask Claire Hooker and Louise Stone in Chapter 3, when the doctors insist that there is *nothing* wrong? In their chapter, the authors examine the nature of the conflicts which produce the psychosomatic, particularly the ways in which the biomedical model skews the balance of power between experts and laypeople. Hooker and Stone study how the discursive construction of diagnostic categories depends greatly on who controls not only "knowledge" but also the central explanatory metaphors of "health" and "illness". Although we tend to take the mechanism of scientific knowledge for granted, Hooker and Stone point out the influence of analogy – and its underlying assumptions – in shaping what we know, or believe we know. A history of unexamined figurative usage inevitably reproduces figurative, biased readings of "facts" – which also necessarily exclude from consideration that which cannot be categorized.

The psychosomatic is often over-simplistically used to obscure complicated social and moral judgments in the reassuring disguise of empirical, biomedical discourse. Taking "good health" for granted, as a marker of the neoliberal subject's ability to manage the burden of "responsibilization" imposed by the ideologies of late capitalism, it then becomes necessary to reread ill-health as a marker of failure. Stress, anxiety, depression are not allowed to be symptomatic of a disorder in culture. Rather, we tend to revert to pseudo-Freudian assumptions of unresolved, specifically individual neurosis, that, if repressed in the psyche, manifest in the individual body as various "somatic" symptoms. Thus, the psychosomatic can always be a medicalizing explanation that never yields to medical treatment, a symbol whose actual referent cannot be confronted, and must be displaced to the responsibility of the suffering individual. In Chapter 4, in her history of emotional eating in twentieth-century American culture, Jessica Parr describes exactly this problem, where requirements about economically productive and gender-normative behavior became inextricable from emerging theories about the mind and body, as centered specifically on the medico-moral judgment of fatness. As Parr explains, research advancements in physiology and metabolism were less culturally effective in explaining overweight than psychological, psychoanalytic assumptions about overeating as a psychosomatic symbol for unresolved problems of identity and emotion.

From these more specific studies of the psychosomatic's problematic application in the biomedical model, in Chapter 5, Amba Sepie moves to a broader epistemological critique, focusing more specifically on the problem of biomedicine as a cultural assemblage which facilitates the diffusion of knowledge and power in culture. Sepie argues that biomedical practices have had a colonizing effect on the discourses of "health," privileging what is knowable and amenable to taxonomy within the constraints of Westernized, scientific inquiry. The psychosomatic defies knowability, even as its persistence and frequency militate for recognition. The problem, Sepie suggests, is Western biomedicine's rigid adherence to a language of stability. In particular, the reductive insistence on dualism as an explanatory model of the mind's relationship to the body inevitably promotes tension around authority and knowledge, constraining providers' and patients' ability to understand one another, and imposing frustrating limits on how we understand mind and body as disparate entities. In response, Sepie makes a case for a decolonizing, anti-hierarchical subversion of biomedicine, an integrative approach that works with, rather than against, the messy, but rich, signifying potential of the psychosomatic.

In Chapter 6, Seamus Barker and Lorimer Moseley continue this critique, applying specific strategies of reading – namely rhetorical and narratological analysis – to challenge the taken-for-granted, unequal relationships of power and authority which exacerbate the conflicts of the psychosomatic. In their study of the psychosomatic – and of pain in particular – Barker and Moseley observe that dualistic, biomedical readings are doomed to failure because of an underlying assumption that disease can only be explained through narratives of coherence and causality. These, in turn, demand clearly delineated claims to agency by the central characters. In the dominant medical narratives encoded in the "bible" of psychological diagnosis, the *Diagnostic and Statistical Manual of Mental Disorders*, agency belongs to the officially sanctioned authors of diagnosis, healthcare providers and researchers; the narrative of the psychosomatic might be *about* the passive sufferers – the patients – but not *by* them. In a discourse which insists on causality, linearity, coherence, and literality, there can be little to no space accorded to the story of the psychosomatic as individuals live it.

If the discourse of biomedicine denies the confounding narrative of the psychosomatic, that does not stop us producing stories about it, and with it. Indeed, as the essays in the second part of this collection demonstrate, the inevitable pull of narrative – as a means by which we all attempt to order the most disordered experiences – gives the psychosomatic much work to do in unexpectedly diverse cultural sites. Insofar as the psychosomatic inhabits a space of ambiguity and resistance within a fraught relationship of mind and body, storytellers can apply its metaphorical potential to illustrate conflicts within the individual's larger psychosocial context. As Sontag (1990) warned, to use illness as metaphor runs the risk that we obscure, rather than illuminate, illness as a physiological process. However, as we are unsure of whether the psychosomatic may be physiological or something else entirely, the resultant figurative work that it does *can* help us better understand other processes, other relationships, through the struggle of individuals to reconcile their identity with the often antagonistic demands of Westernized culture.

Bridging the gap between clinical and lay culture, Maria Tutorskaya (Chapter 7) explores how the ambiguity of the psychosomatic makes it emblematic of individual identity as it is upset and destabilized by rites of passage – specifically the transformation from layperson, to student, to physician. Using autobiographical memoir and fiction as her primary sources, she explains how "medicalstudentitis," or medical students' hypochondria, is a well-documented affliction for those studying to become physicians, and one often dismissed as "all in their head." While the maladies of medical students are largely imaginary, the significance of their resulting distress is not: the symptoms that are brushed off as an unavoidable side-effect of sheer cognitive overload may be read as a kind of symbolic ordeal of initiation, as the individual sheds their affiliation with lay culture, and enters into the mysteries of specialized, esoteric, expert knowledge and responsibility. The anthropologist, familiar with such rites of passage, can observe, define, and make explicit this system of meanings from the position of outside observer. For those undergoing the initiation themselves, narrative, featuring the psychosomatic as metaphor, allows them to order their experiences in ways that provide structure and coherence while allowing the mysterious to remain.

The rite of passage is a plot which imposes uncharacteristic order upon the psychosomatic: this is more the exception than the rule. By contrast, if the inherent instability of the psychosomatic allows it to function as a metaphor in narratives of conflicted identity, its typical course – one that resists order or resolution – makes it well suited to stand in for stories of nonconformity or alienation. In particular, As Olaug Lian, Catherine Robson, and Hilde Bondevik, explain in Chapter 8, the historical stigmatization of all things female (and feminine) as non-adherent to the diagnostic categories and prescriptions of patriarchy has given impetus to medico-moral assumptions about hysteria and neurasthenia from the nineteenth century to the present. When the individual with fatigue, lack of attention to controlling one's emotions, and lack of engagement with one's social obligations is read as "hysterical," their status as invalids becomes conflated with their invalidity (Herndl, 1993); that is, they are not performing their gender in a valid way.

But the hysterical, psychosomatic narrative can be appropriated, its invalidity used as a means of protest and rebellion. As Lian *et al.* find, a range of authors from Flaubert to Gilman to Townsend have exploited the psychosomatic identity as a powerful, if unfortunately necessary, outlet for the woman who does not, and cannot, fit into the prescribed plot of a gendered cultural narrative.

Arguably, within the constraining ideologies of postmodern culture, even the individual who aspires to succeed according to the terms of disciplined, neoliberal subjectivity is constantly threatened by instability and incoherence. This calls into question whether the psychosomatic is better understood not just as a conflict between mind and body, but rather as the inevitable disjunction of individual identity vis-à-vis a disordered culture. Where concepts of wellness, even in the broadest biopsychosocial application, deny inexplicable symptoms and unresolved conflicts – within and between the relationships of body, mind, and social roles – the psychosomatic offers a narrative way out. As Camelia Raghinaru finds (Chapter 9), the psychosomatic lends its metaphorical potential to a variety of nonconformist identities, including that of the man who inhabits an unstable, ambivalent position between cultural dominance and marginalization. In her psychoanalytic reading of *The Sopranos*, she suggests that the "hysterical" symptoms of several characters, particularly the central figure of Tony Soprano, may be interpreted as a symbolic expression of unresolved, neurotic conflicts of identity, specifically relating to (hyper) masculinity, class, and ethnicity in the American culture of late capitalism.

It is the impulse of both the authors and the inhabitants of narrative to strive for coherence and resolution – we all prefer the restitution narrative which has a satisfyingly clear, meaningful ending. But the provocation, and arguably one vital, inescapable function of the psychosomatic, comes from the real possibility that the narrative of chaos is the norm. In the final chapter in this collection, Hannah Tweed explores the problem of uncertainty taken to postmodern extremes where, rather than using the psychosomatic, the narrative *becomes* it. In the novel *Poor Things*, all markers of wellness and wholeness – reliability and stable meaning in particular – become the subject of subversive, destabilizing parody. Not everything is ill or broken; but nothing is whole or fixed either. Tweed's chapter makes an uncomfortable suggestion: if psychosomatic illness is a reminder that entropy – instability, randomness, and dissolution – is the fate of all organisms in literal, lived experience, the psychosomatic, by analogy, gives voice to the suspicion that our social lives, our identities, and our relationships are inescapably entropic as well. The psychosomatic may be the emblematic condition of postmodern existence – the narrative that cannot help but tend towards disorder, uncertainty, and illegibility.

Note

1 For more on the problem of the psychosomatic in the clinical context, see Greco 2012; Lipsitt *et al.*, 2015; Wise and Balon, 2015; Yon *et al.*, 2015; Howman *et al.*, 2016; Murray *et al.*, 2016.

References

Barker, K.K. (2008). Electronic support groups, patient-consumers, and medicalization: The case of contested illness. *Journal of Health and Social Behavior, 49*, 20–36.

Barker, K.K. (2011). Listening to Lyrica: Contested illnesses and pharmaceutical determinism. *Social Science and Medicine, 73*, 833–842.

Barsky, A., Orav, E.J., and Bates, D.W. (2005). Somatization increases medical utilization and costs independent of psychiatric and medical comorbidity. *Archives of General Psychiatry, 62*, 903–910.

Bartlett, F.C. (1932). *Remembering*. Cambridge: Cambridge University Press.

Belling, C. (2006). Hypochondriac hermeneutics: Medicine and the anxiety of interpretation. *Literature and Medicine, 25*(2), 376–401.

Creed, Frances H. (2012). The epidemiology of multiple somatic symptoms. *Journal of Psychosomatic Research, 72*, 311–317.

Dimsdale, J., Sharma, N., and Sharpe, M. (2011). What do physicians think of somatoform disorders? *Psychosomatics, 52*, 154–159.

Dum, R.P., Levinthal, D.J., and Strick, P.L. (2016). Motor, cognitive, and affective areas of the cerebral cortex influence the adrenal medulla. *PNAS*: 9922–9927.

Engels, G.L. (1977). The need for a new medical model: A challenge for biomedicine. *Science, 196*, 129–136.

Farkas, C-A. (2014). The blind men and the elephant: Mediating conflicting views of controversial diagnoses. *Trespassing Journal, 4*.

Frank, A.W. (1995). *The Wounded Storyteller*. Chicago, IL: Chicago University Press.

Greco, M. (2012). The classification and nomenclature of "medically unexplained symptoms": conflict, performativity, and critique. *Social Science and Medicine, 75*, 2362–2369.

Hawkins, A.H. (1999). *Reconstructing Illness: Studies in Pathography*. Indiana: Purdue University Press.

Herndl, D.P. (1993). *Invalid Women. Figuring Feminine Illness in American Fiction and Culture*. Chapel Hill: The University of North Carolina Press.

Howman, M., Walters, K., Rosenthal, J., Ajjawi, R., and Buszewicz, M. (2016). "You kind of want to fix it, don't you?" Exploring general practice trainees' experiences of managing patients with medically unexplained symptoms. *BMC Medical Education, 16*, 27.

Hydén, L-C. (1997). Illness and narrative. *Sociology of Health and Illness, 19*(1), 48–69.

Lipsitt, D.R., Joseph, R., Meyer, D., and Notman, M.T. (2015). Medically unexplained symptoms: Barriers to effective treatment when nothing is the matter. *Harvard Review of Psychiatry, 23*(6), 438–448.

Mitchell, D.T. and Snyder, S.L. (2001). *Narrative Prosthesis: Disability and the Dependencies of Discourse*. Ann Arbor: University of Michigan Press.

Montgomery, K. (2006). *How Doctors Think: Clinical Judgment and the Practice of Medicine*. Oxford: Oxford University Press.

Murray, A.M., Toussaint, A., Althaus, A., and Löwe, B. (2016). The challenge of diagnosing non-specific, functional, and somatoform disorders: A systematic review of barriers to diagnosis in primary care. *Journal of Psychosomatic Research, 80*, 1–10.

Nettleton, S. (2006). "I just want permission to be ill": Towards a sociology of medically unexplained symptoms. *Social Science and Medicine, 62*, 1167–1178.

O'Sullivan, S. (2015). *It's All in Your Head: True Stories of Imaginary Illness*. London: Chatto and Windus.

Ring, A., Dowrick, C.F., Humphris, G.M., Davies, J., and Salmon, P. (2005). The somatising effect of clinical consultation: What patients and doctors say and do not say when patients present medically unexplained symptoms. *Social Science and Medicine, 61*, 1505–1515.

Shapiro, J. (2011). Illness narratives: Reliability, authenticity, and the empathic witness. *Medical Humanities, 37*(2). 68–72.

Shattock, L., Williamson, H., Caldwell, K., Anderson, K., and Peters, S. (2013). "They've just got symptoms without science": Medical trainees' acquisition of negative attitudes towards patients with medically unexplained symptoms. *Patient Education and Counselling, 91*, 249–254.

Stone, L. (2014). Blame, shame, and hopelessness: Medically unexplained symptoms and the "heartsink" experience. *Australian Family Physician, 43*(4), 191–195.

Wise, T.N. and Balon, R. (2015). Psychosomatic medicine in the 21st century: Understanding mechanisms and barriers to utilization. *Advances in Psychosomatic Medicine, 34*, 1–9.

Yon, K., Nettleton, S., Walters, K., Lamahewa, K., and Buszewicz, M. (2015). Junior doctors' experiencing of managing patients with medically unexplained symptoms: A qualitative study. *BMJ Open, 5*(12), e00959.

1 Patients with multiple somatic symptoms and their physicians

At the mercy of a medical system

Caryn Kseniya Rubanovich

There is a disconnect that many people feel exists in modern Western medicine, especially in the relationships between physicians and patients (Charon, 2001). The physician–patient relationship is central to good patient care, and when this relationship is less than successful it results in difficulties and undesirable medical outcomes (Hahn *et al.*, 1994; Ong *et al.*, 1995). While this disconnect is observable throughout the different specialties of medicine, it is especially evident in primary care visits between physicians and patients with multiple somatic symptoms (MSS).[1] Both physicians and patients with MSS note experiencing dissatisfaction, frustration, and confusion in their encounters, and report feeling burdened by their visits (Salmon *et al.*, 2007). Patients with MSS may feel let down and, at the same time, physicians may find patients presenting with MSS difficult to work with, and even dread seeing them compared to their other patients (Barsky *et al.*, 2005; Morriss and Gask, 2009). Clearly, such negative interactions are unproductive (Hadler, 2013). Patients with MSS need the kind of physician–patient relationship and communication that will help them make sense of their complex illness experiences (Roter and Hall, 1993). Nevertheless, multiple barriers make this a difficult goal to achieve.

Narrative medicine is one approach that can help us consider the suboptimal physician–patient interactions. Narrative medicine focuses on the physician–patient relationship in the moment of clinical encounter through a literary lens, zooming in and out of stories, isolating details, patterns, and themes, all of which further illuminate patients' narratives. Narrative medicine emphasizes the importance of listening and its ability to foster physician–patient relationships (Charon, 2001). Listening is instrumental for physicians attempting to understand their patients with MSS's "chaos narratives" (Frank, 1995). Stories of MSS are "chaotic" and hard to listen to because they are confusing, frustrating, disorderly, and lack structure (Frank, 1995; Lask, 1996; Nettleton *et al.*, 2005). MSS are medical mysteries that take on varying forms: headaches, dizziness, aches, fatigue, rashes, stomach disorders, chronic constipation or diarrhea, and weight fluctuations (Farkas, 2013; Roter and Hall, 1993). These symptoms evolve, change, disappear, reoccur, and migrate from one location in the body to another, with "no clear beginning or end" (Nettleton *et al.*, 2005, p. 206). For those who have lived with MSS for long periods of time, it is difficult to follow the plot: "to remember the chronology of visits to clinics, specialists, investigations, and results" (Nettleton *et al.*, 2005, p. 206). The chaos narratives of patients with MSS are upsetting for them, and may be challenging for physicians to comprehend and readily solve (Nettleton, 2006).

While it is helpful to use narrative medicine to begin to understand some of the issues that arise in communication between physicians and patients with MSS, this approach alone cannot fully grasp the underlying factors that dictate these medical encounters. Narratives can never be entirely isolated from their larger context. Thus, deconstructing some of the larger, underlying forces that impact upon these individual physician–patient encounters will help us gain further insight into the challenges of medical encounters for patients with MSS and their physicians (Waitzkin, 1991).

Larger societal forces greatly affect individual physician–patient encounters. Western medicine's overall cultural adherence to a medical system that is heavily ingrained in a restrictive biomedical model of medicine, driven by profit-seeking corporations, may exacerbate the suffering of patients, and complicate matters for physicians. Furthermore, whether physicians are fully cognizant of it or not, their medical education, training, and approach towards treatment may serve as a barrier to care. A dominant biomedical philosophy, without the consideration of psychosocial factors, limits physicians' ability to care for patients with MSS, and may be detrimental when it fails to fully address patients' experiences and needs (Crowley-Matoka *et al.*, 2009). In addition, physicians' resources, time, and autonomy, often dictated by external social entities like the pharmaceutical industry and managed care, can escalate the situation. Furthermore, patients themselves may have been conditioned through their lived experiences to prefer the biomedical model. Thus, patients with MSS, and at times their physicians, are victims of "structural violence"; they are on the receiving end of injustices that result from, and are perpetuated by, biomedical systemic-level beliefs of patient care that influence Western medicine (Farmer, 1996).

Dominant societal-level narratives of medicine, health, and illness mold an individual's understandings of these concepts. In the United States, and other places where Western medicine is predominantly practiced, Rafael Campo notes that "it is difficult to utter the word 'medical' or 'medicine' without automatically thinking of today's dominant anti-empathetic biomedical approach to treating patients" (2005, p. 1009). The biomedical model is the "grand narrative" of medicine, one that is simple, clear, and straightforward, and attempts to reduce every illness to the biological level (Morris, 1998, p. 11). The biomedical model certainly has its merits, and has led to significant benefits. Thanks to discoveries rooted in biomedicine, we can expect to live longer lives: antibiotics wipe out bacterial infections, vaccines prevent diseases from disabling patients' futures, and surgeries remove abnormalities and restore function (Morris, 1998). The biomedical model is successful in many ways, and continues to be the main narrative that doctors and patients follow (Morris, 1998).

Nevertheless, the biomedical approach is just one narrative, and cannot accommodate all patients' experiences. The biomedical model is limited by its underlying assumption that illnesses have clear and objective organic causes that are knowable (e.g. through lab results, imaging, etc.). Even though objective evidence and organic causes are rarely found for MSS, patients still greatly suffer (Barsky *et al.*, 2005; Hadler, 2013). At times, these patients may even be worse off physically and mentally than patients with other conditions (Barsky *et al.*, 2005). Although these patients seek out and use a disproportionately high amount of medical care, they rarely experience productive outcomes, thus leaving them with an unsatisfactory quality of life (Dwamena *et al.*, 2009; Salmon, 2007). Without the necessary objective evidence, the biomedical model becomes a barrier to these patients seeking relief (Morriss and Gask, 2009; Nettleton, 2006).

Physicians are immersed in biomedicine and biomedical ways of thinking from their years as students and trainees (Crowley-Matoka *et al.*, 2009). From their early days of medical education, students and trainees are conditioned to accept a biomedical point of view that translates to their patient care (Roter and Hall, 1993). They learn to focus on measurable numbers and data for guidance and reassurance, incorporate the newest medical developments, and master formulaic and reductionist thinking to accurately diagnose patients (Crowley-Matoka *et al.*, 2009; Roter and Hall, 1993). Medical students learn to categorize and separate physical and psychosocial aspects of health as they solidify mind–body dualist ways of thinking inherent in their training (Have, 1987). Medical students learn to focus on the observable symptoms while dismissing other "subjective" symptoms because they are irrelevant (Crowley-Matoka *et al.*, 2009). If symptoms do not indicate an underlying physical disease or disorder, they may be reattributed to psychological causes or emotional disorders, and referred to "psych" (Gask *et al.*, 2011; Salmon, 2000). This kind of knee-jerk dualistic reaction is unproductive for MSS patients, whose suffering may derive from a mixture of biopsychosocial factors.

Physicians' education and training may not adequately prepare physicians to care for, manage, assess, or support patients with MSS (Morris, 1998; Woodward *et al.*, 1995). Social factors may only be mentioned tangentially in medical education, or left out entirely; thus, when issues such as "work, family life, aging, substance use, and sexuality enter the conversation . . . the doctor often has neither training nor authority" to address them (Waitzkin, 1991, p. 276). Physicians may not have the underlying knowledge or confidence to incorporate psychosocial factors and adopt a holistic approach towards their practice (Crowley-Matoka *et al.*, 2009; Dwamena *et al.*, 2009; Salmon, 2007; Salmon *et al.*, 2007). Thus, physicians are at a disadvantage in their medical encounters with patients with MSS.

Patients with MSS often present perplexing cases that prove frustrating to physicians who work within a realm of certainties and probabilities aiming to categorize, diagnose, and treat. Physicians may feel helpless when they are unable to relieve their patients' symptoms. Not surprisingly, physicians may be more keen to view MSS as a "transient stage in the diagnostic process" that will eventually turn into something more biomedically palatable (Farkas, 2013, p. 316). Ideally, MSS would turn into something identifiable and treatable with the newest medical discoveries, technologies, surgeries, and drugs (Nettleton *et al.*, 2005). Nevertheless, even in the absence of objective evidence, physicians may turn to somatic treatments based in the biomedical model out of habit, in an attempt to help (Ring *et al.*, 2004; Salmon, 2000; Salmon *et al.*, 2008). Physicians may approach care and treatment with the same "mindset one brings to the treatment of pneumonia" (Hadler, 2013, p. 170). They may try to get rid of the symptoms rather than address psychosocial factors (Salmon, 2007; Dwamena *et al.*, 2009). Unfortunately, by focusing solely on finding a cure for the physical elements, physicians may stray from the patient's needs and fail to adequately address the patient's overall well-being and health (Crowley-Matoka *et al.*, 2009). Patients with MSS "may actually fare less well today than in times when medical knowledge was less developed" (Nettleton *et al.*, 2005, p. 209).

The biomedical narrative has also affected the ways patients with MSS see their conditions (Crowley-Matoka *et al.*, 2009). Patients have grown up seeing physicians for various health needs (e.g. vaccinations, antibiotics, bone breaks). They may have witnessed physicians tracing their pain, sickness, and suffering back to pathological, anatomical, and biological causes (Morris, 1998). Thus, some patients with MSS may see their symptoms as purely physiological in origin (Farkas, 2013). Due to the ways in which they have largely been conditioned to think of treatment, patients gravitate towards somatic treatments such as surgeries and medication (Morris, 1998). Some patients may have received exposure to pharmaceutical marketing that promised them "restitution" – the full alleviation of symptoms and distress – by simply taking a pill (Frank, 1995). Afterwards, these patients may seek out physicians to test and validate their symptoms, get a diagnosis, and then, hopefully receive biomedical treatment such as medication (Morris and Gask, 2009). Even when patients receive these kinds of treatments, they may not actually meet all of the patients' needs (Salmon, 2000; Waitzkin, 1991).

Although MSS and their pathophysiology are not understood well, they continue to be attributed as disease in Western medicine's reductionist framework (Isaac and Paauw, 2014; Salmon, 2007). With a plethora of makeshift diagnoses available, physicians can categorize MSS into disorders and syndromes such as irritable bowel syndrome, chronic fatigue syndrome, chronic pelvic pain, chronic fatigue syndrome, or fibromyalgia. The somatic syndrome disorders outlined by the American Psychiatric Association for the DSM-5 (2013) are also available, but are lackluster. The diagnoses function as little more than placeholders used to account for symptoms "which have no other obvious or measurable medical cause" (Farkas, 2013, p. 324). This is not to say these diagnoses do not exist; rather, "as explanations, they are tautological" (Salmon, 2007, pp. 246–247).

Naming a patient's experience with a diagnosis may offer relief, and could enable access to new information and resources (Nettleton, 2006; Peters *et al.*, 1998; Woodward *et al.*, 1995). A diagnosis can legitimize patients' experience of symptoms and suffering, ensure others see it as real, and help them feel that they are not alone (Salmon, 2000; Page and Wessely, 2003; Woodward *et al.*, 1995). This kind of acknowledgement is important when patients with MSS seek support from friends, family, and physicians (Dwamena *et al.*, 2009; Nettleton, 2006; Page and Wessely, 2003; Salmon, 2000). Without a diagnosis, patients with MSS may not know how best to communicate their illness experiences to others (Woodward *et al.*, 1995). It is unfortunate that patients live in a culture that "demands that illness be diagnosed first before coping can proceed" (Hadler, 2013, p. 209). Furthermore, patients with MSS may desperately want to pinpoint the cause of their misery so that they can access the immediate benefits of biomedicine (Hadler, 2013).

A diagnosis can have a powerful impact upon a patient's life, and labeling may have negative consequences such as behavioral changes, altered social and personal relationships, and experiences of stigma or discrimination (Frances and Chapman, 2013; Page and Wessely, 2003; Woodward *et al.*, 1995). The act of diagnosing perpetuates the cycle of privileging "patients and illnesses that 'fit' into available diagnostic and treatment options" (Crowley-Matoka *et al.*, 2009, p. 1315). Thus, using biomedical understandings to diagnose patients with MSS may actually "serve to intensify the chaos and uncertainty" they feel (Nettleton, 2006, p. 1175).

Patients with MSS experience complex suffering that resists instant fixes, demands patience, and requires additional time from physicians who may not have that luxury (Crowley-Matoka *et al.*, 2009). Given the time-consuming nature of attending to these patients, it may be tempting to fix the situation by simply pre-scribing medication (Hadler, 2013). Unfortunately, when physicians try to relieve their patients' suffering solely through somatic interventions, they circumvent addressing the contributing factors, and may inadvertently perpetuate the patients' suffering and dependence on medical care (Salmon *et al.*, 2007; Waitzkin, 1991). For patients, taking prescribed medications may further reinforce "the need to 'cure' their disease" (Hadler, 2013, p. 175). Medications may help alleviate some of the suffering of patients with MSS, but they should not be the only available options (Henningsen *et al.*, 2007; Komaki *et al.*, 2009; Morriss and Gask, 2009). Unfortunately, patients may not consider or seek out other forms of psychosocial relief (Salmon, 2000). Furthermore, the immediate reflex to turn to medications as part of the biomedical model keeps the pharmaceutical industry thriving (Morris, 1998). As soon as MSS become unnecessarily medicalized and diagnosed, these patients become the next potential "consumers" of the pharmaceutical indus-try looking for quick fixes (Hadler, 2013; Waitzkin, 1991). The pharmaceutical industry is aware of this potential consumer base, and has since tried to establish a "foothold" (Hadler, 2013, p. 174). Regardless of whether prescription medica-tions really are the best treatment option for patients with MSS, they are lucrative for profit-seeking pharmaceutical companies motivated by money.

Researchers and clinicians have also written about the ways in which man-aged care might negatively affect patient care and physician–patient relationships (Crowley-Matoka *et al.*, 2009; Forrest *et al.*, 2002; Hadler, 2013; Morris, 1998). Managed care can frustrate physicians and patients, and make them feel power-less (Morris, 1998). Physicians have expressed concerns about managed care and its effect on their patient relationships (Feldman, Novack, and Gracely, 1998). Instead of feeling like being in partnership with each other, they may feel that their encounters are directed by insurance companies that get in the way of physi-cians' "ethical obligations" (Feldman *et al.*, 1998, p. 1629). Due to the emphasis on constant productivity, and the pressure to see more patients, many physicians feel overwhelmed (Feldman *et al.*, 1998). Without adequate time to arrange productive and comprehensive medical visits, physicians are limited in the care and services they can offer patients with MSS. Patients may feel rushed, and mention the symptoms at the surface level rather than having an in-depth discussion of what they are experiencing. Managed care interferes with the care physicians give and their ability to put the patients' needs first, ahead of other incentives (Feldman *et al.*, 1998). Furthermore, physicians have to work with a system that may reimburse for certain treatments, but not for taking time to fully understand their patients' conditions (Crowley-Matoka *et al.*, 2009). At the end of the day, insurance companies are in the business of making money, and whether the needs and suffering of patients are actually being met may not be a top priority (Crowley-Matoka *et al.*, 2009; Hadler, 2013). In this kind of environment, the physician's autonomy is challenged by "cost-conscious bureaucrats" (Morris, 1998, p. 13). Ultimately, this results in compromised care (Waitzkin, 1991).

From narrative medicine, we see how the power of *being* with another in the medical encounter and accompanying them through their suffering provides relief that must not be underestimated (Charon, 2001). Physicians themselves can be the greatest therapeutic tools for their patients (Balint, 2000). Furthermore, the physician–patient relationship is one of the most important factors for successfully managing patients with MSS (Heijmans *et al.*, 2011). Indeed, it should be "at the heart of the practice of medicine," and "at the center of effective treatment" for patients with MSS (Isaac and Paauw, 2014, p. 669). Nevertheless, if the United States' medical and healthcare systems continue "institutionalizing conflicts of interest," patients with MSS will receive suboptimal care (Hadler, 2013, p. 189). As long as it is in the best interests of certain medical entities to maintain the status quo, and to reinforce the biomedical model regardless of the consequences, physicians' listening and decision-making will be threatened, and patients will fail to receive the genuine care they deserve (Hadler, 2013, p. 11). These aspects of the larger medical system along with the biomedical model of thinking in which physicians are immersed fail to accommodate patients with MSS and reinforce their suffering; they may even perpetuate problems for physicians as well (Hadler, 2013; Page and Wessely, 2003). Physicians themselves are affected because they experience "frustration, anger and burnout" as a result of these barriers, which has severe repercussions for the physicians and their patients (Crowley-Matoka *et al.*, 2009, p. 1320). Finally, as long as the biomedical narrative is dominant, patients with MSS will continue to suffer, since this single narrative inadequately accounts for their symptoms and experiences.

Considering larger social forces exposes many of the limitations of current medicine. Indeed, one goal of this chapter is to encourage both physicians and patients to reflect and see the ways that the biomedical culture in which they are located shapes their expectations and health-related interactions (Crowley-Matoka *et al.*, 2009, p. 1319). Health requires more than a biomedical model of thinking (Engel, 1977; Hadler, 2013). Thus, clinical medicine should address the health continuum by incorporating molecular, social, and psychological factors of health to help patients with MSS (Brody, 1985; Chiapperino and Boniolo,

2014; Engel, 1977; World Health Organization, 1946). By understanding how the dominant narrative of biomedicine is interwoven into Western medicine, we can begin to make the appropriate changes to cultivate a more comprehensive and responsive view of health that would benefit patients with MSS and the physicians who care for them. Even more, this shift may help physicians better support various needs from *all* of their patients. With the help of narrative medicine in conjunction with a systemic-level approach to understanding issues present in physician–patient relationships, the medical community is empowered to recognize its shortcomings, highlight its strengths, and cultivate a well-rounded practice.

Note

1 A literature search of ambiguous somatic symptoms recovers some of the following terms: "'hysteria,' 'dysfunctional,' 'factitious,' 'psychosomatic,' 'somatization,' and so on" (Nettleton *et al.*, 2005, p. 207). Even more, symptoms may be further diagnosed as "psychosomatic disorder," "somatoform disorder," "somatic symptom disorder," and others. The ways for describing ambiguous somatic symptoms has evolved over the past few decades. As terms acquire negative connotations they become stigmatizing and may be retired. The term "medically unexplained symptoms" (MUS) is a commonly used catchall term in the research literature. Originally, MUS was a description of symptoms, but, during the course of its use, MUS became a label (Nettleton, 2006, p. 1168). For the purposes of this chapter, I use "multiple somatic symptoms" (MSS) instead of the term "medically unexplained symptoms" (MUS) (Creed *et al.*, 2012). This linguistic distinction is a conscious decision to use a neutral term (Greco, 2012). Creed and colleagues (2010) point out that "MUS" is a problematic term for the following reasons: (1) it perpetuates dualistic thinking by implying that medically explained symptoms are organic, while medically unexplained symptoms are psychological in nature; (2) it suggests that since symptoms are "medically unexplained," medicine cannot address them; (3) it perpetuates a biomedical model of medicine that does not include psychosocial or cultural factors (Henningsen *et al.*, 2007, p. 947). Knowing how to respectfully describe an individual's experience is a vital part of physician–patient communication, which is a key entry point for the physician–patient encounter (Salmon *et al.*, 1999, p. 372). The other terms previously utilized either hold negative implications or are counterproductive (Greco, 2012; Salmon, 2007). Even these kinds of subtleties are important because they can have profound effects over time.

References

American Psychiatric Association. (2013). Somatic Symptom Disorder. Available at www.dsm5.org/documents/somatic symptom disorder fact sheet.pdf.

Balint, M. (2000). *The Doctor, His Patient and the Illness*. Edinburgh: Churchill Livingstone.

Barsky, A., Orav, J., and Bates, B. (2005). Somatization increases medical utilization and costs independent of psychiatric and medical comorbidity. *Archives of General Psychiatry*, 62, 903–910.

Brody, H. (1985). Philosophy of medicine and other humanities: Toward a wholistic view. *Theoretical Medicine*, 6, 243–255.

Campo, R. (2005). "The medical humanities," for lack of a better term. *JAMA: The Journal of the American Medical Association*, 294(9), 1009–1011.

Charon, R. (2001). Narrative medicine: A model for empathy, reflection, profession, and trust. *JAMA: The Journal of the American Medical Association*, *286*(15), 1897–1902.

Chiapperino, L., and Boniolo, G. (2014). Rethinking medical humanities. *Journal of Medical Humanities*, *35*, 377–387.

Creed, F. H., Davies, I., Jackson, J., Littlewood, A., Chew-Graham, C., Tomenson, B., and Mcbeth, J. (2012). The epidemiology of multiple somatic symptoms. *Journal of Psychosomatic Research*, *72*(4), 311–317.

Creed, F. H., Guthrie, E., Fink, P., Henningsen, P., Rief, W., Sharpe, M., and White, P. (2010). Is there a better term than "medically unexplained symptoms"? *Journal of Psychosomatic Research*, *68*, 5–8.

Crowley-Matoka, M., Saha S., Dobscha, S. K., and Burgess, D. J. (2009). Problems of quality and equity in pain management: Exploring the role of biomedical culture. *Pain Medicine*, *10*(7), 1312–1324.

Dwamena, F. C., Lyles, J. S., Frankel, R. M., and Smith, R. C. (2009). In their own words: Qualitative study of high-utilising primary care patients with medically unexplained symptoms. *BMC Family Practice 10*(1), 67.

Engel, G. L. (1977). The need for a new medical model: A challenge for biomedicine. *Science*, *196*(4286), 129–136.

Farkas, C. (2013). Potentially harmful side-effects: Medically unexplained symptoms, somatization, and the insufficient illness narrative for viewers of mystery diagnosis. *Journal of Medical Humanities*, *34*, 315–328.

Farmer, P. (1996). On suffering and structural violence: A view from below. *Daedalus*, *125*(1), 261–283.

Feldman, D. S., Novack, D., and Gracely, E. (1998). Effects of managed care on physician–patient relationships, quality of care, and the ethical practice of medicine: A physician survey. *Archives of Internal Medicine*, *158*, 1626–1632.

Forrest, C. B., Shi, L., von Schrader, S., and Ng, J. (2002). Managed care, primary care, and the patient–practitioner relationship. *Journal of General International Medicine*, *17*(4), 270–277.

Frances, A., and Chapman, S. (2013). DSM-5 somatic symptom disorder mislabels medical illness as mental disorder. *Australian and New Zealand Journal of Psychiatry*, *47*(5), 483–484.

Frank, A. W. (1995). *The Wounded Storyteller: Body, illness and ethics.* Chicago, IL: University of Chicago Press.

Gask, L., Dowrick, C., Salmon, P., Peters, S., and Morriss, R. (2011). Reattribution reconsidered: Narrative review and reflections on an educational intervention for medically unexplained symptoms in primary care settings. *Journal of Psychosomatic Research*, *71*(5), 325–334.

Greco, M. (2012). The classification and nomenclature of "medically unexplained symptoms": Conflict, performativity and critique. *Social Science and Medicine*, *75*, 2362–2369.

Hadler, N. M. (2013). *The Citizen Patient: Reforming health care for the sake of the patient, not the system.* Chapel Hill: University of North Carolina Press.

Hahn, S. R., Thompson, K. S., Wills, T. A., Stern, V., and Budner, N. S. (1994). The difficult doctor–patient relationship: Somatization, personality and psychopathology. *Journal of Clinical Epidemiology*, *47*, 647–657.

Have, H. A.M. J. T. (1987). Medicine and the Cartesian image of man. *Theoretical Medicine*, *8*, 235–246.

Heijmans, M., olde Hartman, T.C., van Weel-Baumgarten, E., Dowrick, C., Lucassen, P.L.B.J., and van Weel, C. (2011). Experts' opinions on the management of medically unexplained symptoms in primary care. A qualitative analysis of narrative reviews and scientific editorials. *Family Practice, 28*, 444–455.

Henningsen, P., Zipfel, S., and Herzog, W. (2007). Management of functional somatic syndromes. *The Lancet, 369*, 946–955.

Isaac, M., and Paauw, D. (2014). Medically unexplained symptoms. *Medical Clinics of North America, 98*, 663–672.

Komaki, G., Moriguchi, Y., Ando, T., Yoshiuchi, K., and Nakao, M. (2009). Prospects of psychosomatic medicine. *BioPsychoSocial Medicine, 3*(1), 1.

Lask, B. (1996). "Psychosomatic medicine" not "psychosomatic disorders". *Journal of Psychosomatic Research, 40*(5), 457–460.

Morris, D.B. (1998). *Illness and Culture in the Postmodern Age*. Berkeley: University of California Press.

Morriss, R., and Gask, L. (2009). Assessment and immediate management of patients with medically unexplained symptoms in primary care. *Psychiatry, 8*(5), 179–283.

Nettleton, S. (2006). "I just want permission to be ill": Towards a sociology of medically unexplained symptoms. *Social Science and Medicine, 62*, 1167–1178.

Nettleton, S., Watt, I., O'Malley, L., and Duffey, P. (2005). Understanding the narratives of people who live with medically unexplained illness. *Patient Education and Counseling, 56*, 205–210.

Ong, L.M.L., De Haes, J.C.J.M., Hoos, A.M., and Lammes, F.B. (1995). Doctor–patient communication: A review of the literature. *Social Science and Medicine, 40*(7), 903–918.

Page, L.A., and Wessely, S. (2003). Medically unexplained symptoms: Exacerbating factors in the doctor–patient encounter. *Journal of the Royal Society of Medicine, 96*, 223–227.

Peters, S., Stanley, I., Rose, M., and Salmon, P. (1998). Patients with medically unexplained symptoms: Sources of patients' authority and implications for demands on medical care. *Social Science and Medicine, 46*(97), 559–565.

Ring, A., Dowrick, C., Humphris, G., and Salmon, P. (2004). Do patients with unexplained physical symptoms pressurise general practitioners for somatic treatment? A qualitative study. *British Medical Journal, 328*(7447), 1057–1060.

Roter, D., and Hall, J.A. (1993). *Doctors Talking with Patients/Patients Talking with Doctors: Improving communication in medical visits*. Westport, CT: Auburn House.

Salmon, P. (2000). Patients who present physical symptoms in the absence of physical pathology: A challenge to existing models of doctor–patient interaction. *Patient Education and Counseling, 39*, 105–113.

Salmon, P. (2007). Conflict, collusion or collaboration in consultations about medically unexplained symptoms: The need for a curriculum of medical explanation. *Patient Education and Counseling, 67*, 246–254.

Salmon, P., Peters, S., and Stanley, I. (1999). Patients' perceptions of medical explanations for somatisation disorders: Qualitative analysis. *British Medical Journal, 318*(7180), 372–376.

Salmon, P., Peters, S., Clifford, R., Iredale, W., Gask, L., Rogers, A., and Morriss, R. (2007). Why do general practitioners decline training to improve management of medically unexplained symptoms? *Journal of General Internal Medicine, 22*, 565–571.

Salmon, P., Wissow, L., Carroll, J., Ring, A., Humphris, G. M., Davies, J. C., and Dowrick, C. F. (2008). Doctors' attachment style and their inclination to propose somatic interventions for medically unexplained symptoms. *General Hospital Psychiatry, 30*, 104–111.

Waitzkin, H. (1991). *The Politics of Medical Encounters: How patients and doctors deal with social problems*. New Haven, CT: Yale University Press.

Woodward, R., Broom, D., and Legge, D. (1995). Diagnosis in chronic illness: Disabling or enabling – the case of chronic fatigue syndrome. *Journal of the Royal Society of Medicine, 88*, 325–329.

World Health Organization. (1946). Preamble to the Constitution of the World Health Organization as adopted by the International Health Conference, New York, 19–22 June 1946; signed on 22 July 1946 by the representatives of 61 states (Official Records of the World Health Organization, no. 2, p. 100) and entered into force on 7 April 1948.

Further reading

Aiarzaguena, J. M., Gaminde, I., Clemente, I., and Garrido, E. (2013). Explaining medically unexplained symptoms: Somatizing patients' responses in primary care. *Patient Education and Counseling, 93*(1), 63–72.

Barsky, A. J. (1979). Patients who amplify bodily sensations. *Annals of International Medicine, 91*, 63–70.

Dimsdale, J. E., Creed, F., Escobar, J., Sharpe, M., Wulsin, L., Barsky, A. J., and Levenson, J. (2013). Somatic symptom disorder: An important change in DSM. *Journal of Psychosomatic Research, 75*(3), 223–228.

Escobar, J. I., Gara M. A., Diaz-Martinez, A. M., Interian, A., Warman, M., Allen, L. A., and Rodgers, D. (2007). Effectiveness of a time-limited cognitive behaviour therapy type intervention among primary care patients with medically unexplained symptoms. *Annals of Family Medicine, 5*, 328–335.

Fallon, B. A. (2004). Pharmacotherapy of somatoform disorders. *Journal of Psychosomatic Research, 56*, 455–460.

Henningsen, P., and Priebe, S. (1999). Modern disorders of vitality: The struggle for legitimate incapacity. *Journal of Psychosomatic Research, 46*, 209–214.

Janca, A., and Isaac, M. (1997). ICD-10 and DSM-IV symptoms of somatoform disorders in different cultures. *Keio Journal of Medicine, 46*, 128–131.

Kaplan, G., Lipkin, M. Jr., and Gordon, G. H. (1998). Somatization in primary care: Patients with unexplained and vexing medical complaints. *Journal of General International Medicine, 2*, 177–190.

Lin, E. H. B., Katon, W., Von Korl, T. M., Bush, T., Lipscomb, P., Russo, J., and Wagner, E. (1991). Frustrating patients: Physician and patient perspectives among distressed high users of medical services. *Journal of General International Medicine, 6*, 241–246.

Maiden, N. L., Hurst, N. P., Lochhead, A., Carson, A. J., and Sharpe, M. (2003). Medically unexplained symptoms in patients referred to a specialist rheumatology service: Prevalence and associations. *Rheumatology, 42*, 108–112.

Manderscheid, R. W., Ryff, C. D., Freeman, E. J., McKnight-Eily, L. R., Dhingra, S., and Strine, T. W. (2010). Evolving definitions of mental illness and wellness. *Preventive Chronic Disorders, 7*(1), A19.

Rief, W., and Mohan, I. (2007). Are somatoform disorders "mental disorders"? A contribution to the current debate. *Current Opinion in Psychiatry, 20*, 143–146.

Smith, G.R. Jr. (1990). Somatization disorder in the medical setting. National Institute of Mental Health. DHHS Publ. No. (ADM) 90–1631. Washington, DC: US Government Printing Office.

Smith, G.R., Monson, R.A., and Ray, D.C. (1986). Patients with multiple unexplained symptoms: Their characteristics, functional health, and health care utilization. *Archives of International Medicine, 146*, 69–72.

Stanley, I.M., Peters, S., and Salmon, P. (2002). A primary care perspective on prevailing assumptions about persistent medically unexplained physical symptoms. *International Journal of Psychiatric Medicine, 32*, 125–140.

2 Narrative medicine and fibromyalgia

Between facts and fictions, "factions" to be honored

Maria Giulia Marini, Daniele De Nardo, Paola Chesi, and Luigi Reale

Introduction: Fibromyalgia: a real condition or "all in the patient's head"?

What is fibromyalgia? This disease encompasses a variety of symptoms: the most important features are chronic, widespread pain, tenderness in several parts of the body (hands, feet, neck, back), and fatigue. In addition, it may present with sleep disturbances, memory or cognitive dysfunctions, migraine or tension headaches, digestive disease, irritable or overactive bladder, pelvic pain, depression, anxiety, or some combination of these symptoms (Mease *et al.*, 2007; Sarzi-Puttini *et al.*, 2008). For several decades, fibromyalgia has been described under different names and its various sets of symptoms have remained difficult to characterize within a specific clinical category. Only in the past decade has it obtained a name and been recognized as a "real chronic disease" with specific care maps and therapies to improve patients' symptomatology (White and Harth, 2001; Inanici, 2004; Pikoff, 2010; Gillis, 2013).

Patients in the Italian health care system complain that neither physicians nor taxpayers regard this condition with sufficient understanding or consideration. In clinical practice the disorder is still often misdiagnosed, often confused with osteo-arthritis, muscular rheumatism, depression, anxiety, or "hypochondria" (Goldenberg, 2009; Di Franco *et al.*, 2011), putting fibromyalgia in a "twilight zone." This disease is still believed to be "all in the patient's head" and attributed to imagination, often manifesting in people already affected by personal distress (White *et al.*, 2002; Gordon, 2003; Wolfe and Rasker, 2012). Therefore, fibromyalgia continues to be treated as a psychological disorder rather than as a clinical condition. The higher prevalence among females corresponding to a 9:1 ratio, as revealed by Bennet *et al.* (2007), contributes to increase physicians' misdiagnosis of symptoms, interpreted using a gendered approach toward medicine. Physicians' skepticism about symptoms of fibromyalgia seems to be difficult to remove completely, for three main reasons. The first one is that the exact etiology is still unclear, and fibromyalgia is not considered as a clinical entity. The second reason is historical, as the presumed relation between this syndrome and various forms of psychopathology became firmly entrenched in medical culture over a century ago (Hudson and Pope, 1989). Finally, chronic central pain is not a specific topic of study in most medical school programs, with the consequence that health care profession-als still tend to interpret patients' reports of their own pain as a subjective param-eter. Nevertheless, in recent years, some progress has been achieved in defining the diagnosis, in respecting and listening to patients, and in rejecting the stigmatizing connection between fibromyalgia and psychopathology (Yunus, 2008).

However, most patients still often encounter a general preconception or judg-ment from health care providers that they are "not ill" or are affected by "the broken record syndrome." The misdiagnosis of this disease as a mental condition – with possible associated perception that patients are considered *unreliable*, or even *liars* – impacts deeply the quality of the relationship between doctor and those needing care, and represents an obstacle to a proper patient/physician com-munication. People with fibromyalgia who are not understood and believed start a pilgrimage to different centers of care in search of a physician who will listen to them and provide a convincing answer to their condition. Patients' frustration can lead them to repeat tests and examinations compulsively, increasing their lack of confidence in physicians and resentment toward the entire health care system. This "doctor-shopping" phenomenon not only endangers patients' health, it also wastes economic resources both for people with fibromyalgia and for their fami-lies, as well as for the National Health Service.

Because responses to treatment for fibromyalgia vary widely from patient to patient, often with few benefits, physicians may become frustrated in seeing their patients not responding to therapy as hoped.

In the end, treatment of fibromyalgia is frustrating for both patients and their physicians, and the result is that the patient–doctor relationship is severely com-promised by an overall lack of trust due to faulty listening, comprehension, and communication between the parties. In addition, the cultural attitude and stigma-tization of people with fibromyalgia comes from the patients' entire community, as symptoms may affect the sphere of social relationships, causing isolation from family, friends, and colleagues, often leading patients to depression (Åsbring, 2002; Corrigan, 2004; Crooks, 2007; Harakas, 2008; Cohen *et al.*, 2011).

No matter what the etiology of fibromyalgia, a caring and effective social wel-fare system should take into serious account so-called "hypochondriac condi-tions," with the aim to limit individuals' discomfort. Patients' suffering is genuine, and is even exacerbated by the fact that they have to fight to prove the "validity" of their conditions. Patients' journey toward a better "mind" or "body and mind" health status is achieved by taking care of them; this can occur through accurately listening to their needs and perceptions of their disease. As Charon (2006), the founder of the Narrative Medicine movement, explains, the main actions must "honor patients' story of illness" in this "twilight zone" of illness, regardless of whether the narratives are fact or fiction.

A helpful approach: narrative medicine

Greenhalgh and Hurwitz (1998) defined the practice of narrative medicine as "what is circumscribed between the physician and the patient, from the collection of information on events before the disease, to how it has been revealed, focusing on psychological, social and ontological implications." It represents a new tool that can help clinicians connect with patients and gain insight into the disease experience from patients' point of view. The collection and reading of stories told by patients, their families, health care, and social professionals allows the health care team to understand patients' experience with their illness, and figure out the best way to manage their care.

In recent years, many physicians have studied and experimented with narrative medicine, and have testified to how this approach changed their clinical practice by encouraging long-term relationships with their patients, reducing anxiety and insecurities for both patients and professionals, and returning to health care providers a lost sense of care (Charon, 2000; Monsted *et al.*, 2011; Nowaczyk, 2012). Moreover, narrative medicine can be a catalyst for generating sustainability from an economical point of view, as it acts in identifying the most beneficial procedures for the patient, limiting the unnecessary clinical visits and tests so typical in the case of fibromyalgia (Marini and Arreghini, 2012).

Disease, illness, and sickness

The difference between the two terms "disease" and "illness" points to the potential for integration between evidence-based medicine (EBM) and narrative medicine. "Disease" defines the condition from the practitioner's perspective, considered as an objective alteration of the biological structure or functioning and mechanism of the body; "illness" (Kleinman, 1989) refers to the human experience of the physical condition, including the person's perceptions, feelings, and thoughts. While the focus of EBM is on the pathophysiological process, narrative medicine includes the person's judgment and feeling when coping with distress caused by clinical problems (Charon, 2012). Narrative allows both patients and physicians to explore their needs and thoughts which may not be captured by any other means.

A third term to complete the analysis of an individual's experience, *sickness*, refers to how a specific condition is viewed from the perspective of society, "the others." This third point of view includes possible cultural stigmatization and prejudice toward a specific condition, an important element especially in the case of mental or chronic diseases, which can influence the sick person's reactions and behaviors. The term "sickness" is often related to the individual's ability or inability to work, and to their role in relation to social beliefs by and about the ill person (Wikman *et al.*, 2005; Brandt and Rozin, 2013). The trio composed of "disease," "illness," and "sickness" may be used to classify stories of care, to understand the complex relationship among these different components.

Narratives of fibromyalgia

Could fibromyalgia, in the "twilight zone" of hypochondria and the psychosomatic condition, benefit from the narrative medicine approach, using patients' stories as an instrument to improve reciprocal understanding, regardless of whether the disease is considered "real"? Starting in medical school, physicians are educated to believe that data are impartial and objective, and the only medium for telling what is "really" happening in the patient's experience. Driven by an excess of reductionism, this attitude has led physicians to lose their skills of communication and empathy in patient care, as shown by several empirical studies at both undergraduate and graduate levels (Chen *et al.*, 2007; Newton *et al.*, 2008; Hojat *et al.*, 2009).

Consequently, an approach based on patients' narratives is typically met with physician skepticism, as, in their extreme authenticity, such narratives are considered subjective and unreliable, with an outpouring of emotions and colorful descriptions. From a narratological standpoint, it is commonly assumed that "stories are not innocent" (Chambers, 1984), as all of them necessarily contain elements of both authenticity and inauthenticity, and each narrative is always shaped and in some way distorted by the author according to his or her personal choices. Being a blend of facts and fiction, Bury (2001) named stories of illness as "factions." Even when it is clearly not faithful to reality, narrative contains the message the patient needs to express in the moment the story is told. The first-person voice, no matter how incomplete or truthful, still deserves respect and empathy, as it represents the patient's truth in that specific interaction (Shapiro, 2011). Giving such stories dignity and authority provides the foundations for genuine patient-centered care, nowadays a widely over-abused expression but still seldom truly put into practice. Furthermore, narrative medicine is different from the patient's history: the latter is associated with the component of the disease since it consists of a list of body symptoms; narrative medicine treats the realm of illness and, although it can be inspired by real stories, does not necessarily represent daily medical practice.

The parallel chart is a free tool in which physicians write their narratives on patients *with* the history. This extraordinary instrument was defined by Rita Charon (2006), who encouraged medical students and doctors to write about clinical experiences that are not necessarily appropriate in the formal medical record. Physicians' reflective writing on the parallel chart is commonly intended to expose the unique dimensions of patient care. Indeed, it provides a space for physicians to write about the cases they are curing, as well as patients' personal features beyond the mere disease, patients' feelings and outlook, and all the helpful reflective elements for them and their relationships of care.

An experience of the shared patient's diary and the parallel chart

The role of narrative medicine in providing a deeper insight of patients' living with fibromyalgia, toward a long-term physician–patient relationship, has been evaluated in a project performed in Italy in 2012.

Sixteen patients affected by fibromyalgia (1 male and 15 females aged between 30 and 55 years), referring for the first time in an outpatient clinic of a Department of Medical, Surgical and Health Science, were involved. After having signed informed consent, patients were asked to draw up their narrative in a daily diary of their illness, to be shared with the physician, describing their psycho-physical, relational, and emotional state for a period of up to 40 days (from T0 = day 0 to T1 = day 40). Patients' parallel charts were also written by the clinician, with the aim to test the effectiveness of this tool. The physician used this space in his daily practice to collect his impressions on patients after each visit, the quality of the relationship with them and their caregivers, their reciprocal feelings, and other helpful elements to reflect upon the possible strategy of care, both from the clinical and the relational point of view. In this study, only patients' diaries were shared with the physician, while the physician's parallel chart was not shown to patients. The reason for the physician's decision not to share his parallel charts with patients is mainly due to the experimental nature of this project. In 2012, this study represented the first seeds of the use of parallel charts. This experience was the first approach to narrative medicine not only for the physician but also in his clinic; in this pivotal phase, he did not know how this kind of diary keeping might be interpreted by patients, colleagues, and health care managers.

The researchers had access to both the physician's parallel charts and the patients' diaries for a cross-comparative reading of the narrative evolution along the interaction and management of the care plan. The language of the parallel charts and patient diaries was analyzed with transactional analysis, to investigate the evolution of the relationship throughout the theory of ego states. Transactional analysis was studied for the first time by the psychiatrist Eric Berne, who defined this model to study interactions and transactions between individuals (Berne, 1957; Dussay, 1971; Steiner, 1974; Solomon, 2003). In particular, Berne's assumption was that each personality is composed of various parts: the Parent, the Adult, and the Child ego states. These three ego states are respectively connected to the realms of "felt," "taught," and "reflective" thought (Berne, 1961):

- The *Child* ego state is the part of one's personality that is the hub of emotions, thoughts, and feeling "memories" from childhood. Within this state, two further entities can be identified: the *Free Child* ego state (also referred to as the Natural Child) and the *Adapted Child* ego state (which also contains the *Submissive* and the *Rebellious* Child ego states). The Free Child is the side of spontaneous feeling and behavior. The Adapted Child is the part of our personality which has learned to comply with the parental messages. The Adapted Child can turn into a Submissive Child when limited and repressed by the controlling parent, and even escalate into the Rebellious Child ego state if restrictions cause frustration and anger.
- The *Parental* ego state is a set of thoughts, feelings, and behaviors that are learned or "borrowed" from parents or other main models. It is divided into the *Nurturing Parent,* which is nurturing, loving, and permission-giving, and the *Critical Parent,* representing roles, values, and possible prejudices.
- The *Adult* ego state is the balanced side. It is the part of the personality that can process information and knowledge accurately, up to awareness. It is reflective and, when a problem presents, originates solutions based on facts rather than on prejudged thoughts or childlike emotions.

It is assumed that each individual embraces all three ego states as a result of his or her personality development, and that the prevalence of the ego state changes over time (Berne, 1964; Harris, 1973). Writing, in particular, activates the inner dialogue transaction.

Evolutions of the ego states mirror the reciprocal attitudes of sympathy and trust. Narrative interpreted with transactional analysis represents a precious instrument toward the interpretation of how events evolved during the period of care.

How patients narrate their fibromyalgia

The contents of the patient narratives were analyzed, comparing their attitude at the beginning of the relationship with their physician throughout the encounters.

From patients' adaptation to their rebellion

The patients' diaries depicted the scenario of living with the condition of fibromyalgia, starting from the first random symptoms of pain and fatigue, to daily and chronic manifestations of serious impairments. The patients' words describe a common situation of searching for a solution among different specialists, who do not identify their symptoms, and trying various more or less conventional therapies. In addition, a context of lack of comprehension emerges from their family and colleagues, because no one recognizes the extent of patients' pain. Lacking a name for their disease, they are not recognized as either clinically or socially ill, but rather they are considered plaintive, litigious, and hypochondriac. The most common topics throughout the diaries were living with chronic pain, the feeling of daily fatigue, the search for a response from physicians, the consequences for their family and social life, and their inability to work in an efficient way.

The description of pain

"I could not put my feet on the ground, I felt as if I had spikes under my feet"; "I suffer all around my thighs and knees and I cannot climb stairs"; "My hands hurt especially in cold water or when it is windy"; "My shoulder has been hurting since 2009"; "I can lower myself only keeping my back straight, otherwise I feel an electric shock"; "Sometimes I feel pain from the tip of the hand to the tip of the foot"; "My Achilles tendons have been hurting me since I was 25"; "My feet continuously burn"; "Of course I feel pain, my shoulders are injured and my hand often tingles. Do not speak about my knees!"; "I cyclically feel pains which "tour" throughout all my joints"; "Everything started with a pain in my hands, in particular at the level of thumbs"; "My hips hurt more and more frequently"; "I lie on the bed, with a rigid and painful neck. Level of pain: neck 6, back 8"; "I feel pain as if I had been beaten!"

Fatigue during the day and in the evening

"I feel tired and rigid"; "Lots of tiredness!"; "In the evening I feel exhausted"; "What a tiring day!"; "Tiredness, fatigue, in a funk."

The physicians' misunderstanding and skepticism

"My family doctor seemed skeptical but he did not comment"; "My health problems started when I was 20 and they had always been underestimated because of my young age . . ., you are too young to be sick"; I changed my family doctor but the problem still stays"; "My family doctor told me I had arthritis"; "They told me I had a hernia"; "My family doctor blamed my weight and menopause for my pain"; "These pains are diminished by physicians, nobody asked which was the triggering cause"; "My family doctor explained to me that there are women who suffer from this kind of pain, but it is not worrisome and there is nothing to do."

The repercussions upon family life

"My husband says that I am whining as I am always tired, this makes me feel bad"; "In the evening my husband always has to help me to wash up as I am blocked on the seat"; "Some days my daughter had to go to school by bus, as I could not get up for my tiredness."

Difficulties in daily life

"I cannot lift weights"; "When I drive the car my pelvis and back hurt"; "When I take a shower, dress or wash my feet I have to keep my back straight"; "I cannot stand too long, or walk too much, because pain becomes intolerable; this changed my life"; "You are no longer able to open a can"; "I fold the laundry, but I have to stop."

At work

"This morning I was so tired that my primary school students helped me to bring my bag"; "I care for the elderly, I have to wash, dress, and lift elderly people. Sometimes I cannot do the simplest movements"; "When I work my hand hurts and becomes swollen"; "I had to ask for some days off from work because of the strong pain on my feet"; "All my periods of sickness corresponded to absence from work, these are my absences in the last years: from 22/3 to 9/4 2010; from 7/3 to 5/4 2011; from 15/6 to 9/7 2011; from 16/5 to 25/5 2012."

Results from the transactional analysis demonstrate a *Free Child* patient trait, who is asking for help and attention, and who feels vulnerable and scared. Patients appear also as *Adapted* or *Submissive Children* who have had to follow the physicians' considerations for a long period, and who eventually adhere to various care plans. Furthermore, the analysis reveals the patients' feelings of anxiety, help-lessness, and, in some cases, depression. There are also patients who feel angry (though not openly declaring so) about the situation and drift toward the *Rebellious Child* state.

Diagnosis and treatment of fibromyalgia: patients' Critical Parent ego state which moves to the Adult state

In patients' texts it is possible to distinguish two different moments following the first medical visit: the immediate reaction of doubt regarding the diagnosis of fibromyalgia and the suggested pharmacological therapy, and the feedback after some days of therapy, revealing a progressive day-by-day change of attitude toward the physician and therapy.

The initial doubts regarding therapy

"I do not understand why you are telling me I have FIBROMYALGIA! Because I NEVER COMPLAIN, I HATE PEOPLE COMPLAINING! I am not at all DEPRESSED"; "I took pills of X. for 20 days, 30 milligram, as you prescribed to me, but they are not so helpful"; "After our encounter I started taking the pills that you suggested. I have to say that for the first ten days I was in doubt regarding their usefulness"; "I stopped taking drops of C., as they could be the cause of my tiredness."

After the first doubts, the feedback on therapy reveals signs of a new attitude

"The therapy for fibromyalgia is going well, I feel less rigid in the morning. I have to say that I feel a little bit more relaxed compared to one month ago, but I continue to be so tired"; "After 15 to 20 days I started to feel less tired, my muscles are more released and my daughter also sees me more active. Compared to the time before our encounter, I feel more active. I am happy with how it is going on"; "I feel the pain a little bit less severe. These days are a miracle for me!"

Usually these diaries end with *direct or indirect requests to the physician*

"We would like to have a child, but having fibromyalgia I am not sure I would be able to carry on a pregnancy and be a good mother. And I don't know if I can take drugs during the pregnancy. Tomorrow I will see Doctor . . . I hope he gives me something for my tiredness"; "I hope you can help me, so I can live better"; "Still, my feet burn"; "I still hope to improve."

Analysis of these extracts of diaries shows a progression in the ego states. During the first days, patients revealed skepticism regarding diagnosis and therapy, and they tended to deny the effect of their medication, continuing to suffer pain and feeling rigid and tired. From their reflective writing, the *Critical Parental* ego state is revealed, as they are all very judgmental toward the physician, believing themselves to be the only ones who know what they are experiencing, and considering the clinician almost like a child who is getting everything wrong. In some cases they also take on the role of *Rebellious Child*, and decide to interrupt therapy or change something in it, considering themselves more expert than the physician. Yet, day after day, they reveal that they feel better, less rigid, in less pain, and more active. Such relief for this good sensation leads them to change their attitude toward both therapy and physician, and in some cases they start the transition toward the *Free Child* ego state, as they feel astonished and grateful for the improvement. Furthermore, they start to acquire awareness of their condition and reactions to therapy as a first step which could lead them to the *Adult* ego state.

A disease-centered approach

Stylistically, many patient texts resemble a clinical chart more than a diary: such narratives may be considered to be mainly *disease-centered*. There is little space for the *illness* component, with brief mentions about the patients' emotional state and their family and social life. Such dryness in narration is likely explained by the general lack of openness toward their physician, and to the fact that conversations with the caring physician are limited to the clinical aspects. However, deeper analysis suggests an attempt by the patient to communicate with the doctor using his language in order to obtain his attention and comprehension. Importantly, however, patients – after an initial hesitation – generally agreed to write a diary about themselves with the aim of being understood. They showed trust in the narrative process.

How the physician considers his patients

The second step of the study was to analyze the physician's experience of his thoughts and impressions as collected in the parallel charts.

The early Adapted Child ego state

The analysis of the physician's parallel charts confirms the difficulties encountered by health care professionals in managing care for fibromyalgia patients and attempting to find a solution to their suffering. From the first meeting, the charts depict the evolution of a complicated relationship, the (not always successful) attempt to understand patients' symptoms and reach a diagnosis, and the difficulty of continuing a therapeutic project despite the lack of trust and adherence from the patient.

The first approach: patients' attitudes

"She has a worried and suspicious face, accompanied by a funereal friend. Zero trust in physicians, zero trust in medicines. She does not open herself to me. Her

friend looks at me more and more surly"; "This patient is very angry with eve-rything and everybody"; "She is annoyed toward physicians and is very rigid"; "She does not take off her sunglasses"; "She looks at me with a challenging smile"; "She seems a little bit depressed: she does not shake hands with vigor, speaks only a few words, her gestures are limited, makes many grimaces"; "He is very shaken, speaks in a confused way. He is like a flooding river, out of breath while speaking."

Patients' stories of pilgrimage

"She says she has been visiting different physicians for years and she followed a day hospital in hematology without knowing the reason and the result"; "Years and years of investigations"; "I listen to all her misfortunes, she lists in a messy way different physical disturbances"; "He moves from a problem of perspiration, to feet burning, then talks about shoulders and cervical spine. He talks about infil-trations, FANS, cortisone, ultrasound, laser"; "We start to talk about her prob-lems and she starts a real stream of consciousness."

The surplus of examinations

"She gives me a bundle full of documents with zillions of tests from the last three years"; "I see all the tests done over and over again"; "She gives me a bag full of Rx, tests, analyses, certificates made by physiotherapists, orthope-dists, neurologists and therapists from all over the city. She literally pours all these documents on my desk. The first one dates back to 1997! Some exams were repeated up to five times"; "From a bag she extracts an actual radiologic volume and a compendium of laboratory analyses"; "She wants me to look at all her previous exams. My computer starts to grind while uploading all these investigations."

Patients' reaction to diagnosis and proposed therapy

"She already visited four other rheumatologists and all of them gave her the same diagnosis of fibromyalgia, but she always refused to take therapies as she thinks that medicines are 'poisons'. Finally I told her that she has fibromyalgia, and she with a hysterical laugh says: 'Don't you give me the fibromyalgia story too! I am not mad! I am not an imaginary sick person!'"; "She does not appear convinced about diagnosis and therapy, and when I talked about antidepressants, she made a strange face. I explained to her she is not depressed. As she is leaving the room, with every step she stops and tells me a new symptom, right up to grabbing the door handle; I think she is not satisfied with my diagnosis, she is afraid I am missing something"; "I explain to her that her symptoms are not arthritis and she seems to be sorry for this. She already researched everything about arthritis on internet. She says she will do a pelvic X-ray, as if she wanted to say to me 'You will see, I have arthritis'."

At the second visit the physician talks about patients' resistance to
therapy and a continuing skeptical attitude

"I suggest to her a drug but she prefers to carry on with physiotherapy"; "I ask
her if she started to take D and she answers with the face of a child caught with
her hands in the jam, and says she has not yet requested the prescription from her
family doctor. She starts to describe her pain again, she asks me if she has arthri-
tis or whatever. How is it possible, I have already explained fibromyalgia to her
in the previous visit! I explain everything to her over again, using simple words.
Still, as last time, she does not seem convinced"; "Reading her story, I discover
she does not take D . . . she does not trust me!"; "She says to me that nothing
changed and while we complete the test she gives me negative answers before
I finish questions."

Such stories, from the physician's perspective, seem to emphasize his feelings
of helplessness: *"Pressed, disarmed in front of this flood of words, complaints,*
and sometimes delirium"; "In difficulty"; confused: *"HELP! I do not understand*
anything!" The physician feels defeated: *"I wonder if my communication with*
patients is efficient"; "What a failure!"

In examining the physician's words, it seems that there is a sort of inversion
of roles between patients and physician. He feels judged, pressed, not believed
and recognized in his role, seeming an *Adapted Child*, sometimes even a little
scared as a *Free Child*. Patients, on the other hand, are not described as the free or
adapted children we saw across their diaries, but rather recurrently as a *Critical*
Parent ego state; in the parallel chart their judging, suspicious, and even aggressive attitude is emphasized.

The reciprocal mistrust: the physician's Critical Parent ego state

Another important element of mistrust may be found in the physician's words,
with regular expressions indicating skepticism toward patients' oral descriptions
and judgment of the common image of people with fibromyalgia:

"Her pen falls on the ground and she bends down to pick it up . . . didn't she
suffer from backache?"; "She starts to talk about a series of dubious symptoms";
"I pretend to believe her but this is not possible at all"; "She exaggerates her
discomfort in a theatrical way"; "She describes cysts in her feet that, with all my
goodwill, I cannot see, but she describes them as being big"; "I realize that he
is not in such pain"; "She is a strange person with fibromyalgia, not the usual
complaining patient!"; "A colleague of mine referred a boy to me, telling me he
is affected by more psychic than physical problems."

Like his patients, the physician reveals a *Critical Parental* ego state, because
he does not completely believe his patients and considers part of their explanations and gestures as exaggerated and theatrical. This attitude may be partially
explained also by the Italian medical culture, still paternalistic and based on a top-
down relationship, where the physicians generally order the therapeutic strategy

and the patient has to passively obey. However, a process aiming at a concordance between patient and physician, a shared decision-making, still requires time, since it implies a deep cultural change not only in health care professionals but also in patients who are used to considering physicians as the only "acknowledged brain" in the clinical encounter.

In summary, the first part of patients and physicians' stories (T0 = day 0) shows the reciprocal mistrust between the physician and patients, creating obstacles in the relationship of care and the pathway.

Toward a stable alliance: the activation of the Adult ego state

In the second part of the narratives (from T0 = day 0 to T1 = day 40), we can identify the day-by-day transitions of the ego states and an increase of trust and reciprocal understanding. Indeed, in subsequent visits the physician perceives a more relaxed atmosphere as patients are less "threatening", challenging, suffering, and are sometimes even calm and satisfied:

"She seems to be more smiling"; "She speaks more than the last time"; "This time the atmosphere seems less funereal"; "She seems more calm"; "This time she seems more convinced"; "She feels comfortable, unlike last time when she was so rigid"; "She shakes my hands with vigor"; "The patient is satisfied, even if her muscle soreness persists; also her daughter says things are going better"; "She is happy."

At the end (T1 = day 40), the process of building a long-term relationship has been started and the physician is more optimistic:

"There is a hope to set up a calm and efficient relationship"; "She says that I am the kindest physician she has ever met and she has not felt this good in years."

At the end of the process

From the final texts, the Adult ego state has become noticeably developed both in patients and the physician, compared to the first visit. People with fibromyalgia are more aware about their condition and treatment plan, more patient, and open to collaborate for a progression of therapy; the physician is more able to manage the situation thanks to the first results obtained and everyone's changed attitude.

We can sum up the transactions of ego states, clustered over time and connected to the progression of the relationship between patients and physician. At T0 = day 0, the Critical Parent state from patients causes in the physician the activation of the Adapted and Submissive Child state, and, vice versa, the Critical Parent attitude from the physician induces in patients a sense of frustration up to rebellion. After the first encounter and during the writing activity, from T0 = day 0 to T1 = day 40, these ego states diminish over time as new attitudes are activated. Patients feel more comfort in the relationship with the physician, since they are acknowledged for their condition; developing their Free Child state, they are relieved by these first improvements and grateful. On the other hand, the physician acquires knowledge and skills which allow him to leave the initial Submissive ego state and take on a more assertive and determined role capable of providing clear directions to treat fibromyalgia, moving to the Adult ego state. Moreover, his medical skills move in parallel with his empathy, and the clinician accepts from patients every kind of story, even "factions." The physician also activates the *Nurturing Parent* ego state, because he knows the patients' stories better and has established a trustful connection. This transaction has an effect on patients, activating their Adult state as well. Eventually, at T1 = day 40, patients are more relaxed and collaborative during the visits: patients and doctor are both *Free Children*, as now they are more comfortable communicating with one another.

This experience revealed narrative to be helpful in most represented cases. The narratives of the daily building of the relationship between patients and physician end with the activation of the process of alignment. Two main successful elements may be identified to reinforce the relationships of care: the use of narration and the physician's acceptance of patients' stories.

The use of narrative to decrease the "doctor shopping" phenomenon

The patients' diaries activated the transaction from the Critical Parent to the Adult ego state, allowing both to overcome cultural barriers through a process of *decontamination* from stereotypes. The narratives assert that fibromyalgia is not "all in the head," but an illness with clinical impacts upon bodies and lives, which can be treated and managed with the help of a trusting patient–doctor relationship.

The physician's parallel charts also give important feedback on the use of narration. From their initial mistrust toward both the clinician, and the unprecedented detour from clinical protocol, patients were pleasantly moved to write their diaries and share their thoughts with him. Furthermore, they clearly appreciated the opportunity to write a diary, perceiving it as valuable attention from the physician, where they could vent their emotions, have a say in the progression of their condition, and feel listened to: *"She says there was a slight improving of her condition and that her story was useful to her to vent, after years of peregrinations among physicians"; "She says there are few physicians available to listen to their patients' stories."*

After one single encounter, the diaries establish a sort of continuous dialogue between patients and physician, allowing the former to feel more grateful not only for their physical improvement, but also for the impression of being listened to and understood. The physician, reading diaries, sees his own attitudes mirrored back at him, recognizes the weak points, and changes his approach, adopting the best strategy for each patient. In some cases, he acquires precious elements for the diagnosis on patients' condition, personality, and mood that they wouldn't otherwise admit: *"His written story and his tranquility, perhaps because now he trusts me, helped me to reach the diagnosis. What a nice surprise. Thank you narrative medicine!"*

From a methodological point of view, this case shows the possible required "space" of narrative. In an outpatient context where available time is short, narrative generally had to be assigned out of the clinic, representing a tool to continue the dialogue between patient and physician outside the center of care. The physician wrote his parallel charts at the end of the day when visits were over, finding a moment for reflection. Patients, throughout their diaries, wrote about themselves whenever they wished after the visit, and were free to provide more information without the stress of the clinic. During subsequent visits, the moment of sharing stories did not influence the duration of the encounter, but rather contributed to the reciprocal understanding, making the visit more fluid and efficient. The time invested at the beginning of the relationship was gained back during the clinical encounter. As demonstrated in a recent study (Langewitz *et al.*, 2002), narrative medicine does not necessarily require extra time if the whole process of care is regarded. The use of narrative in medicine is mostly an approach based on a more cultural and mental predisposition to listening to and deep understanding rather than a different clinical practice. Therefore, this case may be extended to other clinical contexts and health care professionals, representing a new way of living the profession of health care. Narrative medicine has been successfully applied all over the world in several daily practices, from outpatient visits to intensive care units (Combe, 2005; Griffith and Jones, 2007; Egerod and Christensen, 2009; Vaccarella, 2011; Bødker *et al.*, 2011; www.icu-diary.org).

Regarding parallel charts, the physician recognized the importance of keeping his own texts without sharing them; he used this tool to reflect upon his difficulties with patients with fibromyalgia without any type of censure. What would have happened if the physician's thoughts had been shared? We saw how much the reading of diaries during visits contributed to greater understanding and the establishment of a common point of view. Patients were very honest: at the beginning they clearly admitted to doubts, to be unsatisfied, without trying to please the physician, and all of this was very helpful for him because he could recognize his mistakes and change. However, how useful would it have been for patients to read the physician's comments about them? And how much could this sharing have changed the contents of parallel charts? The physician would probably feel pressured, and less free and open.

The best and most strategic relationship: honoring the "factions"

Independently from the style and content of diaries, the physician made the effort to challenge his own skeptical doubts about his patients' theatrical and exaggerated descriptions, and considered the whole written texts as an important, true source of information and insight into their point of view. What the physician did in this case study, despite his initial skeptical attitude shown during clinical visits, has been called by Das Gupta (2008) an operation of "narrative humility," resisting the dichotomy of real/unreal and the cultural stigma toward people with fibromyalgia. He welcomed any kinds of stories, honoring the "factions," the mixture of factual and perceived elements. Following this process, he realized that fibromyalgia is not just "all in their heads" because at least parts of the narrative are true, and this is enough to understand patients' requests and needs. On the other hand, patients, finally feeling heard, appreciated this form of respect, and became more open to dialogue in response.

Narrative medicine represents a bridge between patients with fibromyalgia and physicians, offering a concrete and efficient strategy to build long-term and constructive caring relationships, combining therapy with narrative and fact with fictions, to honor *factions*. Broadening the horizon up to other "possible hypochondriac conditions" considered by the scientific community or by society as "all in the patient's head," this model of constructive care with narrative medicine has enormous potential. This method is shown to be effective in patients' engagement, with a more satisfying relationship between them and their providers, and with less consumption of resources, by ending patients' "pilgrimage" to find the "ideal" physician. The art of listening and accepting "fictions" is therapeutic by itself and transforms an "ordinary" doctor into an "ideal" doctor.

References

Åsbring, P. (2002). Women's experiences of stigma in relation to chronic fatigue syndrome and fibromyalgia. *Qualitative Health Research, 12*(2), 148–160.

Bennet, R.M., Jones, J., Turk, D.C., Russell, I.J., and Matallana, L. (2007). An internet survey of 2,596 people with Fibromyalgia. *BMC Musculoskeletal Disorders, 8*, 27.

Berne, E. (1957). Intuition V. the ego image. Reprinted from the *Psychiatric Quarterly, 31*, 611–627.

Berne, E. (1961). *Transactional Analysis in Psychotherapy*. New York: Grove Press, p. 4.

Berne, E. (1964). *Games People Play – The Basic Hand Book of Transactional Analysis*. New York: Ballantine Books.

Bødker, S. *et al.* (2011). The use of narratives in medical work: A field study of physician–patient consultations. ECSCW 2011: Proceedings of the 12th European Conference on Computer Supported Cooperative Work, September 24–28, Aarhus, Denmark.

Brandt, A.M. and Rozin, P. (2013). *Morality and Health*. Abingdon, Oxon: Routledge.

Bury, M. (2001). Illness narrative: Fact or fictions? *Sociology of Health and Illness, 23*(3), 263–285.

Chambers, R. (1984). *Story and Situation: Narrative Seduction and the Power of Fiction*. Manchester: Manchester University Press, p. 7.

Charon, R. (2000). Patients and doctors: Life-changing stories from primary care (review). *Bulletin of the History of Medicine, 74*, 871–872.

Charon, R. (2006). Narrative medicine: Honoring the stories of illness. *The New England Journal of Medicine, 355*, 2160–2161.

Charon, R. (2012). At the membranes of care: Stories in narrative medicine. *Academic Medicine, 87*, 342–347.

Chen, D., Lew, R., Hershman, W., and Orlander, J. (2007). A cross-sectional measurement of medical student empathy. *Journal of General Internal Medicine, 22*, 1434–1438.

Cohen, M., Quintner, J., Buchanan, D., Nielsen, M., and Guy, L. (2011). Stigmatization of patients with chronic pain: The extinction of empathy. *Pain Medicine, 12*(12), 1637–1643.

Combe, D. (2005). The use of patient diaries in an intensive care unit. *Nursing in Critical Care, 10*(1), 31–34.

Corrigan, P.W. (2004). Structural levels of mental illness stigma and discrimination. *Schizophrenia Bulletin, 30*(3), 481–491.

Crooks, V.A. (2007). Exploring the altered daily geographies and lifeworlds of women living with fibromyalgia syndrome: A mixed-method approach. *Social Science and Medicine, 64*(3), 577–588.

Das Gupta, S. (2008). Narrative humility. *The Lancet,* 371(9617), 959–1044.

Di Franco, M. *et al.* (2011). Misdiagnosis in fibromyalgia: A multicentre study. *Clinical and Experimental Rheumatology, 29,* Supplementary 69, S104–S108.

Dussay, J.M. (1971). Eric Berne's studies in intuition. *Transactional Analysis Journal, 1,* 34–45.

Egerod, I. and Christensen, D. (2009). Analysis of patient diaries in Danish ICUs: A narrative approach. *Intensive and Critical Care Nursing, 25*(5), 268–277.

Gillis, B.S. (2013). Fibromyalgia, a real medical disease. Available at www.fmcpaware.org/fm-a-real-medical-disease.html.

Goldenberg, D.L. (2009). Diagnosis and differential diagnosis of fibromyalgia. *American Journal of Medicine, 122*(12), S14–S21.

Gordon, D.A. (2003). Fibromyalgia syndrome. *Workplace Safety and Insurance Appeals Tribunal.*

Greenhalgh, T. and Hurwitz, B. (1998). Why study narrative? In T. Greenhalgh and B. Hurwitz (eds), *Narrative Based Medicine: Dialogue and Discourse in Clinical Practice.* London: British Medical Journal Books, pp. 3–16.

Griffith, R.D. and Jones, C. (2007). Seven lessons from 20 years of follow-up of intensive care unit survivors. *Current Opinion in Critical Care, 13,* 508–513.

Harakas, P. (2008). Depressive symptoms, perceived stigma, and perceived social support in fibromyalgia and osteoarthritis patients. *Arizona State University* 33194812008.

Harris, T.A. (1973). I'm ok you're ok. *Library of Congress Catalog Card Number,* 69, 13495.

Hojat, M., Vergare, M.J., Maxwell, K., Brainard, G., Herrine, S.K., Isenberg, G.A., Veloski, J., and Gonnella, J.S. (2009). The devil is in the third year: A longitudinal study of erosion of empathy in medical school. *Academic Medicine, 84*(9), 1182–1191.

Hudson, J.I. and Pope, H.G. Jr. (1989). Fibromyalgia and psychopathology: Is fibromyalgia a form of "affective spectrum disorder"? *Journal of Rheumatology,* Supplementary 19, 15–22.

Inanici, F. (2004). History of fibromyalgia. Past to present. *Current Pain and Headache Reports, 8,* 369–378.

Kleinman, A. (1989). *The Illness Narrative, Suffering, Healing and the Human Condition.* New York: Basic Books.

Langewitz, W., Denz, M., Keller, A., Kiss, A., Rüttimann, S., and Wössmer, B. (2002). Spontaneous talking time at start of consultation in outpatient clinic: Cohort study. *British Medical Journal, 325,* 682–683.

Marini, M.G. and Arreghini, L. (2012). *Narrative Medicine for a Sustainable Healthcare System.* Milan: Lupetti.

Mease, P. *et al.* (2007). Fibromyalgia syndrome. *The Journal of Rheumatology, 34,* 1415–1425.

Monsted, T., Reddy, M.C., and Bansler, J.P. (2011). The use of narratives in medical work: A field study of physician–patient consultations. ECSCW 2011: Proceedings of the 12th European Conference on Computer Supported Cooperative Work, September 24–28, Aarhus, Denmark.

Newton, B.W., Barber, L., Clardy, J., Cleveland, E., and O'Sullivan, P. (2008). Is there hardening of the heart during medical school? *Academic Medicine, 83*, 244–249.

Nowaczyk, M.J.M. (2012). Narrative medicine in clinical genetics practice. *American Journal of Medical Genetics, 158A*, 1941–1947.

Pikoff, H.B. (2010). The psychological mislabeling of fibromyalgia. *International Musculoskeletal Medicine, 32*(3), 129–132.

Sarzi-Puttini, P. *et al.* (2008). Fibromyalgia: Who should reshape the pain perception of these patients? *Reumatismo, 60*, Supplementary 1, 1–2.

Shapiro, J. (2011). Illness narratives: Reliability, authenticity and the empathic witness. *Medical Humanities, 37*(2), 68–73.

Solomon, C. (2003). Transactional analysis theory: The basics. *Transactional Analysis Journal, 33*(1), 15–22.

Steiner, C. (1974). *Transactional Analysis of Life Script*. New York: Grove Press.

Vaccarella, M. (2011). The art of medicine narrative epileptology. *The Lancet, 377*(9764), 460–461.

White, K.P. and Harth, M. (2001). Classification, epidemiology and natural history of fibromyalgia. *Current Pain and Headache Reports, 5*, 320–329.

White, K.P., Nielson, W.R., Harth, M., Ostbye, T., and Speechley, M. (2002). Chronic widespread musculoskeletal pain with or without fibromyalgia: Psychological distress in a representative community adult sample. *Journal of Rheumatology, 29*(3), 588–594.

Wikman, A., Marklund, S., and Alexanderson, K. (2005). Illness, disease, and sickness absence: An empirical test of differences between concepts of ill health. *Journal of Epidemiology and Community Health, 59*, 450–454.

Wolfe, F. and Rasker, J.J. (2012). Fibromyalgia, in G.S. Firestein *et al.* (eds), *Kelley's Textbook of Rheumatology*. Philadelphia, PA: Elsevier, 9th edition, pp. 733–752.

Yunus, M.B. (2008). Central sensitivity syndromes: A new paradigm and group nosology for fibromyalgia and overlapping conditions, and the related issue of disease versus illness. Seminars in Arthritis and Rheumatism. Published online, January 21.

3 Medically unexplained symptoms and the ethics of diagnosis

What does it mean when the doctor says there's nothing wrong?

Louise Stone and Claire Hooker

Case studies

Anna has a two-year history of severe pain in the hand. Multiple investigations have not revealed a diagnosis. Gradually the specialists have withdrawn, with little left to offer. Anna is facing the fact that she may have a long-term disability, with loss of function in the hand, chronic pain, and no way of making sense of either. Many of her family and friends are now questioning her disability, and her workplace is suggesting she may need a different job. At her last consultation, she seems tearful and demoralized, and asks her doctor, "Do you think this is all in my head?"

Dr Anthony Tsau, a young GP (general practitioner, or family physician), has been seeing Miriam Carr for months now. Miriam has been suffering from longterm fatigue, muscle aches and pains, and "weird rashes" which Anthony has not yet seen, because these rashes are fleeting and difficult to capture in a photo. Miriam has tried a number of conventional and complementary therapies, with little change in her condition, and she is angry that no one can provide "an answer" to her distress. Anthony, along with different specialists to whom he has sent referrals, has investigated various serious possibilities, to no end. Finally, Miriam presents with a folder of information she has obtained online, and tells Anthony she has Lyme disease. Miriam asks him to refer her to an international clinic that provides a highly expensive regime of treatment which sounds clinically hazardous. Anthony is concerned about Miriam's well-being, but when he points out that Lyme disease has never been conclusively diagnosed in Australia, and so Miriam needs to be careful, she becomes angry and accuses him of dismissing her needs. "You just think this is all in my head, don't you doctor?"

Caroline is in her sixties and has had a difficult life. A victim of early childhood sexual abuse, she was placed into foster care at a young age and has had a series of relationships with alcoholic and abusive partners. She has a past history of breast cancer, lost one of her children to "cot death," has needed to manage children with mental illness and addiction issues, and is now the primary carer for three of her grandchildren. She presents today to her GP with joint pain. This has been an ongoing issue, and she has had multiple investigations and a series of expert opinions. To date, no one has been able to isolate a cause for her pain. Today, she seems defeated and overwhelmed, and says to her doctor, "My daughter thinks it's all in my head."

Introduction

> Nobody wants an anonymous illness.
>
> (Broyard, 1992)

People who suffer from conditions that are "all in the head" lose the battle for medical legitimacy. "All in the head" is a common construction implying that the illness is "anonymous," imaginary. The phrase has become a default classification for patients who do not fit biomedical diagnostic categories (Jutel, 2010). Illnesses often become "all in the head" at the end of a long and fruitless diagnostic journey, when doctors may withdraw from patient care, feeling they have little to offer once their biomedical taxonomies have failed to be helpful (See Stone, 2014b). Spoken or unspoken, it typically denotes being dismissed and disempowered by health professionals and the health system – even where doctors do not intend this to occur.

In a system of organ-based taxonomy, psychosomatic illness sits uneasily between biomedicine and psychiatry. If symptoms are in the body but the cause is thought to be in the mind, psychosomatic illness sits in the psychiatric taxonomy, and patients are defined – even if they do not experience psychiatric symptoms – as psychiatrically unwell. When doctors can find no biomedical diagnosis, and patients do not accept a psychiatric one, the illness becomes "medically unexplained" (Salmon, 2007). Left in a diagnostic no-man's land, these patients describe fighting for credibility, trying to keep their sense of self intact in the face of a medical narrative that offers little in the way of explanation, treatment, or prognosis (Nettleton, 2006).

As demonstrated by our case studies, there are a variety of circumstances in which illness may appear to be "all in the head" and diagnostic categories have changed over time. Hysteria has become conversion disorder or neurasthenia or somatization disorder, with each psychosomatic illness presenting differently, despite similar presumed etiologies (Shorter, 1992). Nor can we divorce these varying illnesses from the social structures and signification in which they are embedded.

This intersection between medical and social worlds occurs in real time in clinical consultations. We authors are a primary care/family doctor (known in Australia as a general practitioner or GP) with extensive experience both in treating and training other doctors to treat patients with psychosomatic illnesses; and a critical theorist/cultural studies-oriented sociologist of health and medicine. In this chapter, we examine where social theory intersects with primary care for patients with an illness that may be "all in one's head."

Primary care doctors play a prominent part in the lives and experiences of people with symptoms which have little or no basis in underlying organic disease or are out of proportion to existing disease (Smith *et al.*, 2005). Patients with medically unexplained symptoms can experience significant suffering with profound disability, but without a biomedical diagnosis doctor and patient struggle to make sense of the suffering (Nettleton *et al.*, 2004).

What is "real"? The structure of signification in psychosomatic illness

An illness that is "all in one's head" is not considered "real." Psychosomatic illnesses are discursively constructed as deceptive: imaginative projections of the mind that seem like bodily impairments but are not. Pain becomes a mask for the "real" suffering, which is located in the self: in trauma, distress, or even in troubled social power relations. However, since the mind, the will, and the self are paradigmatically conflated, psychosomatic illnesses are seen to be controllable by the minds that created them. With both bodily and psychological symptoms seen as not real, Anna, Miriam, and Caroline become illegitimate as "real" patients with "real" needs. It is therefore not surprising that they are seeking reassurance from their doctors, fearful, clearly, of the answer and what it might signify for their sense of self.

Of course, Anna, Miriam, and Caroline are themselves not "real." They are composites drawn from numerous cases, instantiating three familiar patterns among narratives of psychosomatic illness likely to prompt three different sorts of strategies in clinical management. Through this chapter, the reader can judge how "real" these classifications are.

The "realness" of medically unexplained illness turns in part on how the mind is thought to act on the body to produce physical suffering. In the twentieth century, explanation has predominantly come from psychoanalytic concepts such as sublimation and repression (Lowe *et al.*, 2008). But these explanations do not explain what physical processes may be occurring: the "how" remains mysterious. Contemporary neuroscience is beginning to build better understandings – for example, by showing how trauma affects the neurological system, changing the body's experience of pain and interpretation of stress (Browning *et al.*, 2011). Even so, no well-elaborated mechanism for the mind–body connection has been universally accepted (Sharpe and Carson, 2001).

Mind–body dualism defines the term "psychosomatic" (Sadler, 2004). Thinking of "mind" and "body" as distinct from, and opposite to, each other is deeply embedded in medicine, one of a series of binary oppositions that have structured modern Western thought: male/female, subject/object, active/passive, objective/ subjective, culture/nature, rational/emotional, science/society, among others. These dualisms structure representations of psychosomatic illness. For example, the subject position "doctor" is culturally constructed as rational, unemotional, objective, neutral, and reliable, able to make a scientific assessment that will allow him to validly "know" – through diagnosis – what is wrong with the patient. The subject position of a patient is defined by the other half of these oppositions: invalid (indeed, in-valid), passive, immanent, irrational, and unreliable, a body to be "known." It is easy to see how Anna, Miriam, and Caroline get positioned in this way, even as they and their GPs navigate a more complex relationship. Psychosomatic illness is partly seen as illegitimate because in decoding the patient's subjective experience, the doctor's direct observation as a way of knowing is privileged (Greco, 2012; Sullivan, 1986). Something for which this biomedical "gaze" cannot account (Sharpe and Mayou, 2004) must be considered as "not real."

In biomedical discourse, the term "psychosomatic" reifies these dualisms, constructing them as a fact of nature, so much assumed that they become invisible (Stahl, 2016). In theoretical terms, reification describes the process by which social relations, generated and distributed in capitalist economies, come to be understood as objective realities: the "thingification" of social relations. Reification is a long-running theme in the history of psychosomatic illness, perhaps most infamously in the concept of "hysteria," which naturalized particular views of women's capacities and place in society (Gilman, 1993). We emphasize that the various constructions of "psychosomatic illness," including various biomedical formulations, can and should be theorized as products of the cultural relations of late capitalism, not the experiences and suffering of people in themselves.

What is "real" is constructed through a series of dilemmas in primary care

Anna, Miriam, and Caroline seek, desire, and fear their doctors' authoritative decision as to whether their physical suffering is actually "all in my head." Doctors must ask themselves the same question. Such patients present a series of dilemmas for doctors (Stone and Gordon, 2015) which are intrinsically and inescapably ethical, and simultaneously ontological, epistemological, sociological, and political (Sadler, 2004, 2005). Doctors worry about these patients: is my patient's pain "real"? Or is it better thought of more as an artifact of the brain? Should I order invasive tests to ensure that I do not miss a serious diagnosis, or is that just treating my own anxiety around "missing something"? Will tests merely expose the patient to the risk of iatrogenic harm for no real purpose – or worse, entrench in patients the expectation that disease will inevitably be unearthed with another expensive and potentially harmful investigation? Can we be sure that there is no damage to these patients' bodies that is causing their physical suffering, even if existing tests find nothing (Dimsdale and Dantzer, 2007)? And the ultimate chicken-and-egg dilemma: is their depression a result of unremitting and effectively untreatable suffering, or is it actually the cause of the illness?

Many doctors will find it difficult to even identify the basis for answering these questions. Psychiatrists, GPs, and physicians are committed to staying close to what is real. They are clinicians, not philosophers. In fact, they may feel that it is particularly important that they define what is "real" for patients who may have psychiatric illness and therefore have difficulty making judgments about reality. A diagnosis of some category of psychosomatic illness may be the best description of reality that a doctor has, and hence becomes a very important, if imperfect, standard.

Dilemmas of the real are instantiated in diagnosis

These dilemmas crystallize through the act of diagnosis – indeed, in the question of whether Anna, Miriam, or Caroline can be "diagnosed" at all. Is one of these patients more amenable to diagnosis than the others? The patients themselves seek diagnosis: it offers validation (Nettleton *et al.*, 2004), diminishes the pain and fear of uncertainty (Charmaz, 1983; Frank, 1997), and provides a way forward in choosing therapies and actions (Stone, 2014a). It fits with our Western expectations of illness narrative. For patients, this implies that an illness name leads to an explanation, and hopefully a remedy and restoration to health (Frank, 1997). For the doctor, the narrative is just as powerful: diagnosis leads to evidence-based treatment and then to cure (Stone, 2014a). This "restitution narrative" is culturally expected; it gives the doctor clear direction about how to respond to the patient, what to ameliorate, and when to counsel patience. It gives doctors a rationale for patient care, and the patient a rationale for suffering.

But any of these patients may immediately reject a diagnosis of psychosomatic illness. They may need to hold on to a self-concept as someone who is "normal," not "mentally ill"; they need reassurance that they cannot delete their pain by an act of sufficiently strong will. Their doctors may have additional reasons to refrain from offering such a diagnosis: concern for the stigma their patient may encounter in the medical profession and in the community, for example. Anna is less likely to receive workplace support with a diagnosis of "somatization" than that of "arthritis." Doctors also worry that diagnosis is itself inadequate. Any diagnostic act for Caroline seems to minimize the deep trauma she has endured and survived; yet a diagnosis of "trauma" may entrench her sense of powerlessness. Is it best to know that Caroline's suffering is a product of her trauma, her emotional distress? Or does to "know" this in itself constitute one more moment when the expertise of academics and doctors takes over such a patient's voice (Werner and Malterud, 2003)?

GPs are entrusted to provide care that attends to the patient's unique needs, but at the same time utilizes evidence-based guidelines that guard against observation bias and confirmation bias on the part of both doctor and, to some degree, patient. These are strong motivators that commit GPs to identify what is "real" for these patients, for which diagnosis provides the most significant (and determining) tool.

Naturalistic classification: diagnosis approximating reality

The tasks of medicine are grounded in taxonomy: in scientific classification (Sadler, 2005). "Taxonomical" diagnoses should be rigorous, reliable, and create a valid interpretation of the person's experience; they should provide a sort of shorthand, capturing the essence of the disease with its etiology (cause), prognosis, and characterization (Sadler, 2005).

So when we say "psychosomatic illness," what diagnostic category do we mean? There are, and have been, many options, including somatization disorder, hysteria, neurasthenia, hypochondriasis, conversion disorder, and now somatic symptom disorder. Psychiatric models (such as somatoform disorder), included in the *Diagnostic and Statistical Manual of Psychiatric Disorders* (*DSM*) may involve symptoms in only one organ or organ system, while others occur across multiple systems. Some of these diagnoses imply a psychological cause for physical distress (such as conversion disorder); others try to be etiologically neutral. Some diagnoses are descriptive and intended to imply neither cause nor explanation: one of the most common of these is "chronic pain." Apart from psychiatry, there are diagnoses in other specialties that describe syndromes – clusters of physical and psychological symptoms (e.g. chronic fatigue, irritable bowel syndrome, tension headache). In some cases the consulting doctor may keep the two elements of physical and psychological separate, and diagnose co-morbid conditions (e.g. depression and migraine, anxiety and tachycardia). A doctor may find none of these categories sufficiently satisfactory as to offer a diagnosis. In this case, he or she may simply describe these patients as "medically unexplained": an etiologically neutral term that effectively sidesteps the question of what is "real."

Classification is a difficult act: there are questions as to whether there are sufficient physical, psychological, or social features common to these patients to meaningfully group them as a class (Jutel, 2010). GPs know that these patients commonly present in general practice, and experience significant suffering. Not all patients have multiple or disabling symptoms, but many do; as many have other medical or psychiatric illnesses, or substance misuse (Lowe *et al.*, 2008; see also Stone, 2014a). These patients spend a considerable amount of time accessing health care, often committing to a "career of hospital attendance" (references in Stone, 2014a, 2015). Most are women and many of these patients are victims of childhood trauma (Katon *et al.*, 2001). There is often a history of poor relationships with doctors (Dumit, 2006), and doctors do often find them frustrating to manage (Stone, 2014a).

Given the spectrum from psychiatrists who diagnose somatoform disorders, to GPs who sense "something" similar across different patients, to anti-psychiatry critics of medicalization who see nothing more than social performance in psychosomatic illness (Gilman, 1993), we think it worth the reader's while to pause and consider their own views on the ontology of nosology (disease classification). Classification is always heuristic, a short cut that can stand for reality (and be predictive), but is not itself real; nonetheless, it is intended to capture some aspect of reality. The classifications "leg" and "waist" seem valid; they capture something real: your leg is a different entity to your waist. Yet, if one considers how interconnected muscles and nerves are, reaching up to the shoulder, and down past the knee, leg, and waist become harder to distinguish; harder still if seen primarily as part of the systems of breathing and digestion, of the network of nerves and neurons. Similarly, GPs and patients must confront the "edges" of diagnoses, and distinguish when someone "is" depressed, versus when they are suffering "from" depression, or when "depression" morphs into "anxiety."

Medical classification has often been derived from botanical taxonomy; in that tradition, we can restate the challenge in botanical terms. Consider with what validity we distinguish the 39 species of "lavender" currently formally classi-fied. Some species may be sufficiently similar that they should really be grouped together, or perhaps new distinctions are emerging that may constitute a fortieth species. Or perhaps we are misclassifying "outliers," cases with unusual or dis-proportionate features – like a four-leaved clover or a lavender bush the height of a tree. The criteria one might use to thus "split" or "group" may be phenotypical (that is, the way the plant looks), but they may also be conceptual, such as ecologi-cal niche, or nutrient use, or resilience to shifts in habitat parameters, or evolution-ary history. Precision – that is, how predictably different classifiers will all agree on a classification – should map closely to accuracy, the degree of correspondence between a class and the true state of the thing classified.

So, classification orders knowledge, creating stable and predictive classes that may then be used to seek relationships between classes, refine descriptions, relate individuals to populations, and facilitate future research for so long as the classi-fication is meaningful (Jutel, 2011). However, our classification criteria will "see" some things but hide others: for example, if we classify lavender species by vari-ations in size and shape, we may not even "see" variation in ecological role, let alone recognize it as important.

In medicine, diagnosis is the defining mode of classification. But this is more complicated than botany, because diagnosis is both a set of categories and a social process, and the two are entangled. Diagnosis is key to how medicine creates order (Jutel, 2011; Nettleton, 2006). Epistemically, diagnosis identifies and labels diseases; it specifies treatment, predicts outcomes, and provides an explanatory framework that makes disease understandable. It is easy to reify these diagnostic categories: that is, to forget their heuristic status, and allow the cultural anxieties and social structures that were part of the criteria that formed them to disappear from view.

These are the issues that cluster around the American Psychiatric Associa-tion's *Handbook of Diagnosis, DSM-5*, an object that in itself entangles practice, philosophy, research methodologies, and complex semiosis in public and popu-lar cultural discourses. The *DSM*'s status and influence give it extensive power (Sadler, 2005). Because it offers a common language and standard criteria for the classification of mental disorders, it is used by both patients and clinicians, and orders the systems and organizations that form the structure of health care, from insurance companies and pharmaceutical regulators, to researchers and legal systems (Radden, 2002).

In fact, we could probably diagnose Anna, Miriam, and Caroline by using the two major diagnostic manuals, *DSM* and the WHO-produced *International Classification of Diseases* (*ICD*). Miriam's cluster of symptoms matches with chronic fatigue (*ICD*) and/or depression (*DSM*). Caroline might be diagnosed with depression, somatic symptom disorder, or complex PTSD (a contested diagnosis not found in *DSM* but in common use to describe the cluster of symptoms secondary to childhood trauma). The *ICD* may be called upon to provide a medical rather than a psychiatric diagnosis – in Anna's case, a provisional diagnosis of Morphoea, a condition causing localized thickening of the skin.

Other doctors may critique these diagnoses. For example, they would point to the gap between the criteria used for classification in *DSM*, and the symptom range, quality, and clustering that doctors actually observe in patients (Dimsdale *et al.*, 2009). They may object to diagnoses that are made categorically, rather than in terms of distributions and dimensions (Manning, 2011). Given the substantial overlap between somatoform disorders and depression, anxiety, substance use disorder, and personality disorders, some view these diagnostic categories as "nothing but arbitrary loci in multidimensional space" (Kendell and Jablensky, 2003).

How these diagnostic choices express etiology – the cause or origin of illness – is yet another question. The conceptual roots of these diagnoses may be found in earlier *DSM* taxonomies. *DSM* -III used psychoanalytic theories to ground their classification systems in processes such as conversion, dissociation, or somatization; symptoms were interpreted to be a symbolic expression of intra-psychic conflict (Lowe *et al.*, 2008). *DSM* -IV and -V attempted to be etiologically neutral, and therefore relied on the "objective" process of counting physical symptoms to define psychosomatic disorders, describing a threshold number and types of symptoms. *DSM* -IV also used a multi-axial system of diagnosis that categorized psychiatric diagnosis on one axis and medical diagnosis on another. Where and how to "see" a symptom or a patient remained in debate. Some researchers and clinicians suggested that medically unexplained symptoms be treated as physical diseases with psychological elements in Axis III, rather than psychiatric disorders in Axis I (Mayou *et al.*, 2005). Mayou suggested we code physical symptoms on Axis III and associated psychiatric symptoms would be treated separately as co-morbid conditions (Mayou *et al.*, 2005). And indeed in *DSM*-5, Axis I (principal psychiatric disorder), Axis II (personality disorder), and Axis III (medical or neurological disorder) have been combined, with comments on psychosocial context and functional disability (formerly Axes IV and V) now being considered separately.

For GPs, one way to deal with these challenges is to construct diagnoses in three categories: a medical diagnosis, a psychiatric diagnosis, and a psychological formulation (Stone, 2012). For Anna, this would be a provisional medical diagnosis of Morphoea; a psychiatric diagnosis of possible depression; and a psychological formulation that identifies her demoralization and despair secondary to chronic, overwhelming pain, and her feelings of grief, loss, and isolation. Miriam, by contrast, would be considered for a medical diagnosis of chronic fatigue syndrome, probably post-viral; a psychiatric diagnosis of possible depression; and a psychological formulation of fear and anger due to the lack of an acceptable explanation for her distressing symptoms. There remain sociological questions about the relevance and effect of generating a diagnosis of "depression" so frequently and about what would happen if it just wasn't possible to offer a medical diagnosis (e.g. for Miriam) at all. And indeed, for the GP, the delicacy of these choices is precisely the point, and instantiation, of good care.

These tripartite diagnoses still perpetuate mind–body dualism. Similarly, the continued existence of a category for psychosomatic illness, within the psychiatric classification system of *DSM*-5, still implies that there is a disordered mind producing disordered bodily symptoms. According to one commentator, this represents the fundamental problem in the whole category of psychosomatic illness: "somatisation is a form of convenient terminological wallpaper that papers over the unsightly crack in our understanding of the relationship between mind and body" (Sharpe, quoted in Rosendal, 2005, p. 8).

Diagnosis and power in biomedicine

We have wondered above about the ethics of diagnosing Caroline with depression instead of making the defining feature of her diagnosis be her experience of trauma. Caroline's family may interpret a diagnosis of depression as implying that she also has less responsibility for her suffering: to possess a disease is to be somewhat possessed by it, to imagine the body as active, and the self and the will passive. Caroline may in fact hold two different thoughts at once: a desire to insist on her emotional suffering, while at the same time welcoming a disease-based legitimation of her physical experience. Or perhaps she might care only about whether her GP will now prescribe something that may make a difference in her weary life.

Diagnosis creates access (Jutel, 2009, 2010). It is the key to the status and power of medicine – as the unwillingness of radiographers, nurses, and paramedics (among others) to offer any comment that could be construed as diagnosis attests to today. Diagnosis organizes illness. By determining an explanatory framework, diagnosis determines treatment options and sets expectations for outcomes. Diagnosis has many practical impacts too. It determines the administration of care within a complex health care system, decides who "deserves" care, and structures the professional relations within that system (Jutel, 2009).

For the patient, diagnosis is all-important in three dimensions. The first is the degree of legitimation it grants to the patient's experience, and how that is constructed in the patient's sense of self. Diagnosis has a major role to play in how we "make ourselves up" (Hacking, in Pickersgill, 2014). It segments and orders the patient's very sensations, guiding what should be noticed or ignored, and what stance they should take in relation to their own bodies (Jutel, 2011). This explains why the stakes are so high – nothing less than one's very self – in accepting or rejecting a proposed diagnosis, and why any of our three patients may react angrily to the diagnoses offered. Diagnosis also enables the social incorporation of the patient (Jutel, 2009). It clarifies what society accepts as normal and what is to be regarded as deviance (both in physiology and social action), but incorporates the afflicted person such that they are treated rather than blamed for their deviance (Jutel, 2010; Varul, 2010). This in turn influences the degree and quality of social status or stigma and hence social support that the patient will experience. The third dimension, obviously in interactive influence with the other two, is that diagnosis determines or mediates access to resources such as sick leave, sickness benefits, specialist opinions, and other resources for medical care.

GPs are often very concerned about the social implications of diagnosis for patients like Miriam and Caroline, regardless of their views about the ontology of disease. Often doctors will withhold a diagnosis of somatic symptom disorder or one of its close relatives, purely so that their patient will not encounter stigma, disbelief, and discourteous treatment elsewhere in the health care system (Stone, 2013b, 2014a). Doctors take into account the patient's likely reaction to the diagnosis. In some cases, a diagnosis might offer a welcome legitimation of suffering, and confirm that symptoms are not a projection or distortion of their own anxieties and perceptions. But in others, this knowledge may impede health-seeking behaviors or be used to exercise control in family dynamics, with negative outcomes.

Ambivalence and uncertainty: diagnosis in the social relations of late capitalism

For many doctors, patients like Miriam and Caroline are "heartsink" patients –the doctor's heart sinks when they show up in the waiting room. The doctor has difficulty identifying a naturalistic diagnosis (a medical diagnosis), which is often combined with difficulty in providing appropriate psychological support, in an emotionally challenging consultation. Thus, despite considerable investments in time and concern, doctors often feel they cannot make much of a difference (Stone, 2014a). It is easy for doctors to expect that their attempts to help and support should be met at least with appreciation, not opposition or rejection of a carefully thought-out diagnosis.

The implicit expectations of certain forms of reciprocity in medical consultations are a critical part of how doctors and their "heartsink" psychosomatic patients navigate diagnosis. Patients and their doctors may struggle with diagnostic choices – rejecting the notion that physical pain may be an expression of emotional distress, while simultaneously being haunted, or perhaps even validated, by this possibility (Nettleton, 2006).

But although the experience is deeply personal for each patient, what happens in a clinical interaction is also the product of and a contributor to the social structures and systems of late modernity. Anna's, Miriam's, and Caroline's, and their doctors', navigation between deviance and disease, and the way in which they use diagnosis to construct selfhood (the "good doctor" self as well as the patient selves), are inseparable from the ways in which selfhood is constructed amid the swiftly increasing inequality and insecurity that are features of contemporary society.

As a concept, psychosomatic illness has often been understood as not real in a specific way. Rather than being "ill," patients are expressing and coping with the social stresses that accrue as a result of the demands of self-regulation and performance in highly inequitable capitalist societies (McDonald and Wearing, 2013; Sloan, 1996). One of the most significant such theorizations was Talcott Parsons' concept of the "sick role," which suggests that most illness has psychosomatic elements, since all are motivated by the desire to step back from the performances required by capitalist societies, and to access attention and care instead (Varul, 2010).

Parsons theorized capitalist society as producing and requiring a web of reciprocal role performances, in order to accrue the approval and esteem that organize capitalist societies (Varul, 2010). The sick role is an accepted temporary withdrawal from the burdens of stressful modern life, but the patient is reciprocally obligated to actively seek recovery, and to be compliant with medical advice. Hence doctors' frustration with "heartsink" patients, who do not fulfill the reciprocal obligations of the sick role at all, and whose life narratives similarly do not fit the achievement values and discourses of individual personality and esteem that are built into capitalist cultures (Varul, 2010). In diagnosis, the reification of suffering as disease makes the social relations which produce that suffering invisible, while simultaneously constructing recovery as the moral obligation of the individual.

The point of the sick role as a form of social control is that it manages the deviance of illness on a strictly temporary basis. But for patients with chronic illnesses, especially those likely to persist endlessly, like Caroline's, this may result in the simultaneous demand to conform both to the sick role (in which the "job" of recovery becomes a lifetime employment) and to normal role performances such as caring for children. In this situation, over-compliance with either set of demands – by resting, for example – results in deviance (and failure) from the other (Varul, 2010).

Patients whose illnesses may be "all in their heads" thus embody the social ills of late capitalist, neoliberal "risk" society (Nettleton, 2006). The situation of irreducible and unrelenting "embodied doubt" in an unreliable body and the constant ambivalence (sometimes "embodied paranoia") that patients with complex, enigmatic, or chronic illness may feel toward medicine are hallmarks of post-industrial life (Nettleton, 2006). Miriam's dedication to a diagnosis of Lyme disease – an attempt to take reflexive responsibility for "organising" her illness and "managing" her body by conducting her own health research and then implementing the appropriate bodywork needed for recovery – may be read as mere conformity to the norms of risk society.

Diagnosis is focused on the individual and renders much of the social, cultural, political, and semiotic structures that produce illness invisible. Fixing social inequality or opposing political and power regimes are not part of medicine, though doctors treat the results of both. Nonetheless, doctors, like their patients, may sometimes "see" these issues during clinical interaction. Arguably one primary vehicle for this is narrative.

From botany to gardening: narrative and diagnosis in a therapeutic relationship

Of course, what Anna, Miriam, and Caroline bring to their doctors are their narratives. Patient narratives typically greatly exceed the diagnoses into which they are transmuted. Indeed, the distance from narrative to diagnosis is often taken to stand in for the distance from "illness" to "disease," where "illness" is the subjective experience prior to, and separate from, classification (Woods, 2011; Bolaki, 2016).

While this is a problematically dualistic construction in itself (Bolaki, 2016; Woods, 2011), it resonates with doctors who are struggling to provide care for their patients by means of diagnoses that perpetually fall short of adequately describing patient experiences. In the absence of diagnoses, doctors construct explanations that attempt to position the patient as suffering, but also capable of recovery (Salmon, 2007; Stone and Gordon, 2015). It is a delicate and complex process; they must also recognize, and often subvert the dominant metanarratives available to patients that are unhelpful or destructive to the patient's sense of self. Arthur Frank's tripartite classification of patient narratives – "restitution," "chaos," and "quest" – continues to be recognizable by many patients and doctors (Frank, 1997), though "chaos" narratives of various textures and forms may now be the dominant form in the insecurities of increasingly complex chronic illness and equally complex health and social services (Nettleton *et al.*, 2004; Varul, 2010).

We can at this point reveal the typology behind Anna, Miriam, and Caroline (we did have one). They represent three categories of medically unexplained illness, which we have termed enigmatic illness, contested illness, and chaotic illness (Stone, 2015). Anna represents enigmatic illness. Her symptoms suggest that there is a physiological diagnosis to be made, which cannot be determined at this time (Stone, 2015). If a diagnosis is found, this will transform Anna's illness into a restitution narrative, legitimizing her suffering and probably resulting in the helpful redistribution of tasks at work and at home. Caroline exemplifies chaotic illness – what Arthur Frank terms troubles that are "too complex in both medical and social terms for fixing" (Frank, 1997). Miriam has a chaos narrative too, but she seeks restitution by identifying with a medically contested diagnosis. As Yiannis Gabriel notes, "while stories can be vehicles of contestation, opposition, and self-empowerment, they can also act as vehicles of oppression, self-delusions, and dissimulation" (in Woods, 2011).

Perhaps Miriam would like her illness and her narrative to conform to Frank's third type of illness narrative, namely the "quest" narrative, in which the sufferer is able to transform their suffering by finding meaning in their illness experience. Miriam's "Lyme disease" may provide a battleground (the consultation), a hero (Miriam and the Lyme disease community), and a villain (the medical profession).

Quest narratives are suited to the construction of the "entrepreneurial" self produced by risk society (Nettleton, 2006). However, because her diagnosis is contested, there is a risk that she and her doctor will become enmeshed in the battle for a preferred disease name. It is easy for doctors and patients to be embroiled in a battle over who is right, rather than what is helpful.

GPs cannot pause long to deconstruct these narratives. Instead, they can become fodder for therapeutic engagement (White, 2011). Given the limitations of "botany," or diagnostic classification, doctors and patients often resort to explanations, rather than diagnoses, to provide a framework for care. Such "storied" explanations are often co-constructed by doctors and patients, using and critiquing tropes drawn from the societies in which they live (Stone, 2014a).

These narratives are personal, but may use categories and concepts accepted in the community. For example, this allows her doctor to engage with Caroline in ways that recognize her trauma without constraining her role. Whether the construction is "stress" ("perhaps your body is trying to tell you something") or other folk diagnoses or categories ("adult survivors of childhood abuse," or "victims of domestic violence"), these categories suggest approaches to treatment, potential communities of support, and most importantly, a source for legitimacy (Salmon, 2007).

The great resource for such a GP is metaphor: and such a GP may like to follow Sadler and see this sort of narrative diagnosis as a form of "gardening." "Gardening" involves understanding context (the relations of plants to each other), and usually some form of theme (much like we would describe an English country garden, a Japanese garden, and so on) (Stone, 2013a). This construction allows GPs to explain important therapeutic ideas to patients: recognizing the patient as genuinely ill while working to prevent over-treatment and over-investigation. The important concept behind "gardening" is that it is a collaboration: between experts of various sorts, and the owner of the garden. Successful gardening, like successful collaboration, relies on ongoing interaction and adaption over time.

For those living with an unexplained illness in the precarious environment of contemporary late capitalism, the GP is tasked not so much with diagnosis (much less cure), but with a kind of companionship and a co-creator of meaning–navigating the textures of the chaos over time. Diagnoses may emerge, diagnostic systems may change, and patients may develop other conditions and contexts that alter their needs. Nevertheless, the ability to work across the artificial dichotomy between "body" and "mind" is essential if patients and doctors are to address the complexity of "psychosomatic" illness.

Conclusion

Empirical research, our own and others', has identified that when doctors treat patients like Miriam or Caroline, they worry a lot about whether or not they are being a good doctor (Stone, 2014; Stone and Gordon, 2015). They worry about boundaries: how often they should provide appointments whose primary function is emotional support, when they should judge the clinical relationship as sliding into dependency. They worry that they need to assume "ownership" of a mixed basket-case of suffering, simply because a shuttling journey through the health system has provided no coherency and continuity of care, and yet they feel thoroughly unequipped to do so by virtue of the limitations of billing codes and other structures in the cost-rationing management of health care systems.

The ethics of diagnosis are instantiated in the nuances and complexities of the relationship between doctor and patient. This requires a lot from both parties: the ability to tolerate the discomforts of the relationship and the uncertainty inherent in both the physical and the social situation, not to mention, for the doctor, a kind of reflexive self-confidence with respect to building and navigating appropriate boundaries and suggesting or advocating against particular approaches to treatment. This is a very different stance from the norms that construct a "good doctor": naturalistic diagnosis, and "evidence-based medicine." At worst, it can leave doctors and their patients floundering in an unfamiliar landscape without a map. Nevertheless, the work of the botanists in classifying uncertainty and the work of the gardeners in building narrative fragments and metaphor are essential if patients like Anna, Miriam, and Caroline are to receive the care they deserve for the suffering they undoubtedly experience.

References

Bolaki, S. (2016). *Illness as Many Narratives: Arts, Medicine and Culture*. Edinburgh: Edinburgh University Press.

Browning, M., Fletcher, P., and Sharpe, M. (2011). Can neuroimaging help us to understand and classify somatoform disorders? A systematic and critical review. *Psychosomatic Medicine, 73*(2), 173–184.

Broyard, A. (1992). *Intoxicated By My Illness: And Other Writings on Life and Death*. New York: Ballantine Books.

Charmaz, K. (1983). Loss of self: A fundamental form of suffering in the chronically ill. *Sociology of Health and Illness, 5*(2), 168–195.

Dimsdale, J.E. and Dantzer, R. (2007). A biological substrate for somatoform disorders: Importance of pathophysiology. *Psychosomatic Medicine, 69*(9), 850–854. doi:10.1097/PSY.0b013e31815b00e7.

Dimsdale, J., Creed, F., and Diso, D.-V.W.S.S. (2009). The proposed diagnosis of somatic symptom disorders in *DSM*-V to replace somatoform disorders in *DSM*-IV – A preliminary report. *Journal of Psychosomatic Research, 66*(6), 473–476. doi:10.1016/j.jpsychores.2009.03.005.

Dumit, J. (2006). Illnesses you have to fight to get: Facts as forces in uncertain, emergent illnesses. *Social Scientific Medicine, 62*. doi:10.1016/j.socscimed.2005.06.018.

Frank, A.W. (1997). *The Wounded Storyteller: Body, Illness and Ethics*. Chicago, IL: University of Chicago Press.

Gilman, S. (1993). *Hysteria Beyond Freud*. Los Angeles: University of California Press.

Greco, M. (2012). The classification and nomenclature of "medically unexplained symptoms": Conflict, performativity and critique. *Social Science and Medicine, 75*(12), 2362–2369.

Jutel, A. (2009). Sociology of diagnosis: A preliminary review. *Sociology of Health and Illness, 31*(2), 278–299.

Jutel, A. (2010). Medically unexplained symptoms and the disease label. *Social Theory and Health, 8*, 229–245.

Jutel, A-M. (2011). Classification, disease and diagnosis. *Perspectives in Biology and Medicine, 54*(2), 189–205.

Katon, W., Sullivan, M., and Walker, E. (2001). Medical symptoms without identified pathology: Relationship to psychiatric disorders, childhood and adult trauma, and personality traits. *Annals of Internal Medicine, 134*(9 Pt 2), 917–925.

Kendell, R. and Jablensky, A. (2003). Distinguishing between the validity and utility of psychiatric diagnoses. *American Journal of Psychiatry, 160*(1), 4–12.

Lowe, B., Mundt, C., Herzog, W., Brunner, R., Backenstrass, M., Kronmuller, K., and Henningsen, P. (2008). Validity of current somatoform disorder diagnoses: Perspectives for classification in *DSM*-V and ICD-11. *Psychopathology, 41*(1), 4–9.

Manning, N. (2011). *DSM*: A view from sociology. *Personality and Mental Health, 5*, 112–121.

Mayou, R., Kirmayer, L.J., Simon, G., Kroenke, K., and Sharpe, M. (2005). Somatoform disorders: Time for a new approach in *DSM*-V. *American Journal of Psychiatry, 162*(5), 847–855.

McDonald, M. and Wearing, S. (2013). *Social Psychology and Theories of Consumer Culture: A Political Economy Perspective*. London: Routledge.

Nettleton, S. (2006). "I just want permission to be ill": Towards a sociology of medically unexplained symptoms. *Social Science and Medicine, 62*, 1167–1178.

Nettleton, S., O'Malley, L., Watt, I., and Duffey, P. (2004). Enigmatic illness: Narratives of patients who live with medically unexplained symptoms. *Social Theory and Health, 2*(1), 47–66.

Pickersgill, M. (2014). Debating the *DSM*-5: Diagnosis and the sociology of critique. *Journal of Medical Ethics, 40*, 521–525.

Radden, J.H. (2002). Psychiatric ethics. *Bioethics, 16*(5), 397–411.

Rosendal, M., Per Fink, F.B., and Olesen, F. (2005) Somatization, heartsink patients, or functional somatic symptoms? Towards a clinical useful classification in primary health care. Scandinavian Journal Of Primary Health Care, *23*(1), 3–10.

Sadler, J.Z. (2004). Diagnosis and anti-diagnosis. In J.H. Radden (ed.), *The Philosophy of Psychiatry: A Companion* (pp. 163–179). New York: Oxford University Press.

Sadler, J.Z. (2005). *Values and Psychiatric Diagnosis*. New York: Oxford University Press.

Salmon, P. (2007). Conflict, collusion or collaboration in consultations about medically unexplained symptoms: The need for a curriculum of medical explanation. *Patient Education and Counseling, 67*(3), 246–254.

Sharpe, M. and Carson, A. (2001). Unexplained" somatic symptoms, functional syndromes, and somatization: Do we need a paradigm shift? *Annals of internal medicine, 134*(9), 926–930.

Sharpe, M. and Mayou, R. (2004). Somatoform disorders: A help or hindrance to good patient care. *British Journal of Psychiatry, 184*, 465–467. doi:10.1192/bjp.184.6.465.

Shorter, E. (1992). *From Paralysis to Fatigue: A History of Psychosomatic Illness in the Modern Era*. New York: Free Press.

Sloan, T.S. (1996). *Damaged Life: The Crisis of the Modern Psyche*: Hove: Psychology Press.

Smith, R.C., Gardiner, J.C., Lyles, J.S., Sirbu, C., Dwamena, F.C., Hodges, A., and Goddeeris, J. (2005). Exploration of *DSM*-IV critieria in primary care patients with medically unexplained symptoms. *Psychosomatic Medicine, 67*(1), 123.

Stahl, T. (2016). Georg [György] Lukács. In E.N. Zalta (ed.), *Stanford Encyclopedia of Philosophy* (summer 2016 edn). Stanford, CA: Stanford University Press.

Stone, L. (2012). On botany and gardening: Diagnosis and uncertainty in the GP consultation. *Australian Family Physician, 41*(10), 795–798.

Stone, L. (2013a). Being a botanist and a gardener: Using diagnostic frameworks in general practice patients with medically unexplained symptoms. *Australian Journal of Primary Health Care*, *19*, 90–97.

Stone, L. (2013b). Reframing chaos: A qualitative study of GPs managing patients with medically unexplained symptoms. *Australian Family Physician, 42*, 501–502.

Stone, L. (2014a). Blame, shame and hopelessness: Medically unexplained symptoms and the "heartsink" experience. *Australian Family Physician, 43*, 191–195.

Stone, L. (2014b). Managing the consultation with patients with medically unexplained symptoms: A grounded theory study of supervisors and registrars in general practice. *BMC Family Practice, 15*(1), 1–15. doi:10.1186/s12875-014-0192-7.

Stone, L. (2015). Managing medically unexplained illness in general practice. *Australian Family Physician, 44*(9), 624.

Stone, L. and Gordon, J. (2015). Learning to provide patient-centered care with patients with medically unexplained symptoms: A grounded theory study in Australian general practice. *International Journal of Person Centered Medicine, 4*(3), 173–179.

Sullivan, M. (1986). In what sense is contemporary medicine dualistic? *Culture, Medicine and Psychiatry, 10*(4), 331–350.

Varul, M.T. (2010). Talcott Parsons, the sick role and chronic illness. *Body and Society, 16*(2), 72–94.

Werner, A. and Malterud, K. (2003). It is hard work behaving as a credible patient: encounters between women with chronic pain and their doctors. *Social Science and Medicine, 57*(8), 1409–1419.

White, M. (2011). *Narrative Practice: Continuing the Conversations*. New York: W.W. Norton.

Woods, A. (2011). The limits of narrative: Provocations for the medical humanities. *Medical Humanities,* October, *37*(2), 73–78.

4 Feeding your feelings

Emotional eating in mid-twentieth-century America

Jessica Parr

The metaphorical use of "emotional eating" is pervasive in popular culture. The relationship between emotions and eating is often invoked to explain why we overeat and for approaching weight control in dieting culture. While this psychosomatic explanation for overeating has been increasingly questioned by biomedical research, popular culture has continued to promote the emotional dimension to overeating.[1] It is the origins, the popularization of emotional eating, and the disparity between the popular and medical narratives concerning obesity that will be the focus of this chapter.

The Biggest Loser franchise is perhaps the most recent and well-known mainstream representation that utilizes the emotional eating metaphor. The iconic reality television show seamlessly blends commercialized dieting rhetoric of emotional eating with pseudo-scientific ideas regarding the psychology of weight loss. Other documentaries that present a more scientific method similarly include discussion around the role of emotions in overeating. For example, the three-part British Broadcast Corporation (BBC) documentary *What's the Right Diet for You?* (2015) presented a study investigating the latest weight loss theories related to biochemistry, psychology and genetics. The purpose of the three-part series was to test the most successful weight loss method with the participants being split into three main groups to evaluate three recognized weight loss approaches. The groups were known as the "Feasters", the "Constant Cravers," and the "Emotional Eaters."

Print media also periodically revisit the idea of emotional eating, especially in relation to the obesity epidemic. Major newspapers discuss "emotional hunger" and the lack of an effective strategy to combat this aspect of the obesity problem. In February 2016, the Australian Broadcast Corporation (ABC) published the report "Emotional eating fuelling Australia's obesity epidemic, psychologist says" (2016) claiming that 83 percent of overweight or obese Australians were emotional eaters and expert psychologists urged a mental health approach toward obesity treatment alongside the simplistic "eat less, exercise more" message. There are also a considerable number of examples in health-related periodicals, online blogs, and self-help books that deal with the subject of emotional eating, with the majority of these popular sources directed at a female audience. In general, the discourse presents criteria as to what constitutes emotional eating, often in the form of quiz questions or personal stories to help the reader self-diagnose. Further details are then provided on the cause and a health expert will usually be employed to recommend simplified strategies that can be implemented by the lay-person to help address their emotional eating.[2]

Throughout the twentieth century, the explanation given for the mechanics of weight gain has been the idea of a positive energy balance; the energy ingested through diet and absorbed by the body being greater than the energy utilized by the body. By the 1930s, this energy equation explanation was applied to all cases of obesity (aside from a small percentage of patients with endocrine diseases). The solution recommended by medicine was a reduction in dietary calories and an increase in physical activity to correct the imbalance in energy and facilitate the reduction of body mass. However, further clarification was required to account for excess food consumption, and psychiatry, enjoying increased status due to wartime success, proposed a more complex explanation of why we ate more than our bodies needed. The basic premise, first promoted in the 1940s, was that the root cause of obesity lay in unresolved psychological problems. When confronted with life's challenges the internal psychic conflict experienced by the individual was temporarily subdued with the emotional gratification provided by food. While obesity research challenged the psychoanalytic orientation for overeating in the 1970s, moving toward behavioral, biochemical, and genetic theories, the figure of the emotional eater and what they represented remained in popular culture, developing more complete elucidations to absorb the rise of the behavioral model.

To examine the durability of the emotional eating metaphor in popular culture and explore the variation between popular and medical discourse, this chapter will begin by tracing the origins of the psychological model for obesity to ideas attributed to mid-twentieth-century psychiatry. The convergence of psychoan-alytic and psychosomatic threads in obesity research in the United States of America (USA) during the 1940s presented a new way to consider overeating. The relationship between mind and body in understanding why we overate was negotiated primarily through the role food played in self-regulating feelings of anxiety which, by the 1950s, were believed to stem from deeper psychological problems rooted in childhood experiences. Further, this psychoanalytic-based theory was popularized and disseminated by mainstream periodicals and lay-administered dieting communities in the middle decades of the twentieth cen-tury. The process of popularization and the diffusion of the emotional eating theory in American culture throughout the 1950s will be analyzed in the second and third sections of the chapter, including discussion of the social movement of weight loss groups, one of the most widespread lay-responses to obesity, which utilized the psychology of obesity. The group approach for losing and managing body weight flourished in the postwar USA, promoting emotional eating to a widespread audience and establishing many weight loss practices that still have relevance within contemporary dieting culture today. The chapter will conclude by considering the disparity that exists between popular and medical discourse on the topic of emotional eating.

Medicine

In the 1940s, obesity was increasingly understood in psychoanalytic terms with this theory reaching peak saturation in the 1950s. Prior to the 1940s, the field of endocrinology had classified obesity as an endocrine malfunction. In this understanding, obese persons suffered from an abnormality of the glands which affected their metabolic function, and it was believed that this accounted for their abnormal increase in body fat. However, scientific studies in the 1930s began to show that the great majority of fat people had normal metabolisms and that increased body mass was due to disproportionate calorie consumption in relation to energy expenditure. It was shown that a negative calorie balance would result in a reduction of body weight even in patients who actually suffered from endocrine disorders. In addition, thyroid hormone drugs, often prescribed to treat obesity, were found to be harmful and this helped reduce support for the endocrine approach (Newburgh, 1931, 1942; Bruch, 1939a; Danowski and Winkler, 1944; Rasmussen, 2012). By the 1940s, the decline of "gland-blaming" as a likely explanation for obesity and the general understanding that a restricted diet would produce a reduction in body weight shifted the medical focus to the mechanisms of hunger and appetite. It was at this theoretical intersection, in the 1940s, that medical professionals shifted away from biological approaches to obesity and psychiatry put forward a psychological explanation as to why people overate and frequently struggled to maintain weight loss.

A principal physician in the development of the new psychological theory for obesity was Hilde Bruch, a German-born paediatrician, who immigrated to the USA in 1934 to escape anti-Semitism (Dawes, 2014). Starting in 1939, Bruch published a series of influential studies on childhood obesity that introduced a psychosomatic dimension to the condition. Bruch focused her research not only on the behavior of the children but also on the "family frame" in an attempt to deduce common family environmental factors that may account for why certain children were prone to excessive eating and the avoidance of physical activity (Bruch, 1939b, 1939c, 1940a, 1940b, 1941, 1943; Bruch & Touraine, 1940). From this primary research Bruch concluded that, central to the obese family constellation was a domineering mother who compensated for her own neuroses and her inability to give her child real love by being overly attentive in her role as mother. To the fat child, "food becomes his weapon against anxiety and source of comfort in periods of emotional stress" (Bruch, 1948, p.80).

The psychoanalytic connection between obesity and problematic child rearing, especially in relation to the mother, expanded on "toxic mother" psychology. This connection between overprotective mothering and problematic child development was given scientific legitimacy by the reports of mental health experts in the late 1930s and 1940s (Levy, 1941). According to Bruch, dominant mothering often involved overfeeding and limiting the opportunities of the child for physical activity. The combination of excess food, lack of movement, and a constitutional deficiency in the child resulted in the creation of a passive and dependent child who was unable to discharge urges in a satisfactory manner. Thus, once the child was exposed to rejection or failure he or she was unable to cope and resorted to instant oral gratification as an unfailing source of satisfaction and comfort. To the obese child, food represented the love that was not adequately given by the parents.

Bruch was not a trained psychoanalyst when she first devised her theory concerning childhood obesity. She had personal experience with psychoanalysis in dealing with her own depression. Bruch had also been exposed to the American strands of psychoanalysis and psychosomatic medicine through counsel she sought from colleagues at Babies Hospital in New York, where she had conducted her early obesity research (Dawes, 2014). Bruch did eventually train as a psychoanalyst in the late 1940s but her work on the psychology of obesity was an example of practical psychoanalysis that involved the integration of psychoanalytic, psychosomatic, and environmental intellectual influences that often downplayed the role of sex drives and orality theory, and reduced the use of classic Freudian terminology (Hale, 1995; Dawes, 2014). The central theme of mother blaming and the absence of traditional Freudian terminology were two areas of Bruch's childhood obesity research that provoked contention within medicine. Ironically, the emphasis on toxic mothering and the moderate use of Freudian terminology did predispose her research to popularization, evident in the best-selling book *The Importance of Overweight* in 1957.

Bruch's research was significant in promoting the psychological dimension of obesity and there was a surge in studies published after 1940 by mental health professionals that supported and expanded the psychoanalytic theory. In general, as Rasmussen (2012) has related, further research into the psychology of obesity proposed additional layers to the neurotic personality and tended to apply psychosomatic ideas to an adult population through the analysis of case studies. Psychiatrists Reeve (1942), Richardson (1946), Schick (1947), Hamburger (1950) and Burdon (1951) focused on the mind-body connection presented in the case studies of predominately obese women. They argued that obesity should be considered a symptom of underlying pathology in adults, a case of oral satisfaction beyond socially accepted forms where patients demonstrated a release of tension, a defence mechanism or a compensation for a frustrated libido or frigidity. For example, the clinical research of Hamburger (1951) analyzed the interrelationship between appetite and a person's emotional state, categorizing emotional overeating into four main subgroups: overeating in response to non-specific emotional tension, overeating for gratification in intolerable life situations, overeating as a symptom of underlying emotional illness, and overeating as an addiction to food. Hamburger proceeded to elaborate on the four categories by relating them in simple terms to the psychoanalytic concept of orality with a brief discussion of the possible psychosocial and non-psychological in overeating.

Other psychiatrists, with a greater allegiance to psychoanalysis, further entrenched the psychology of obesity in a psychoanalytic frame by placing more emphasis on conventional Freudian theories (Bychowski, 1950; Rascovsky et al., 1950). According to Bychowski (1950), neurotic obesity was a case of "autoplastic materialization" where the person, in response to challenging circumstances, used the body as a medium for expression. To Bychowski, "Neurotic obesity in women is an autoplastic manifestation of various unconscious impulses and ego-defences" (1950, pp. 318–319). Further, he argued that this involved an increase in early fixations, due to frustrations related to maternal or paternal love objects, producing a trend toward masculinization, and the physical expression of size or a defense mechanism that denied femininity and prevented heterosexual love relationships.

The legitimacy of the psychoanalytic theory in obesity research started to wane in the latter half of the 1960s as psychoanalysis came under general attack from competing medical fields. The fundamental criticism of the scientific credibility leveled at psychoanalysis (Hale, 1995) was also challenged in the research conducted into obese patients treated with both individual and group psychotherapy (Moore *et al.*, 1962; Goldblatt *et al.*, 1965; Penick *et al.*, 1971; Stunkard and Levitz, 1974). Compounding the shift in theoretical sentiment was the lack of practicality which the psychoanalytic model for obesity had offered. The elitist and time-consuming methods of psychotherapy presented little use to the general practitioner who saw the majority of obese people who chose to seek medical help (Kaplan, Kaplan and Leder, 1957; Dwyer *et al.*, 1970).

In contrast to other lifestyle diseases, obesity did not mesh easily with the standard clinical encounter. The intensive talking therapy and support required to address the emotional disturbances of the patient, and to monitor dietary restrictions, were not conducive to primary care. As a result, the treatment prescribed still remained a calorie-reduced diet often with an encouragement to increase moderate exercise and, in many cases, a course of anorexigenic drugs (Kaplan *et al.*, 1957; Rasmussen, 2015). Medicine was also struggling to reform the image of the apathetic doctor who was far from objective in treating their obese patients, characterizing them as "weak-willed," "ugly," and "awkward" in comparison to their thin counterparts (Dwyer *et al.*, 1970, p. 276).

The decline of psychoanalysis and related psychosomatic medicine in obesity research and the rising popularity of behavioral psychology in the 1970s moved the focus in obesity treatment from internal conflict to maladjustment to the external environment. The behavioral model rested on the belief that people overeat as a response to conditioned learning, environmental stimuli, or as a coping mechanism to external stress. Behavioral therapy would often involve methods such as stimulus control, cognitive reconditioning, and forms of behavior modification that aimed to alter the behaviors that were identified with overeating. These treatment approaches allowed a greater degree of standardization in research and a more practical approach in weight control programs.

Popularization

The psychoanalytic theory for obesity did not become the leading approach in general medicine during the postwar years but it did contribute to the establishment of a psychological dimension and the inclusion of mental health professionals in obesity treatment. However, I would argue that the popularization of emotional eating in the 1950s, based on 1940s psychiatric ideas around obesity, was compelling, widespread, and part of the broader extension of therapeutic agents into the American domestic scene after the Second World War (Herman, 1995; Hale, 1995). While the professionalization and growth of psychiatry helped spread the ideas of psychotherapy, it did not solely create a mass demand for psychological services. As Herman has argued, the willingness of the American public to embrace psychological explanations and therapeutic interventions for common medical problems was not only due to the extension of mental health services but also "because it meshed easily with cultural trends that made therapeutic help appear acceptable, even inviting, to ordinary people at mid-century" (Herman, 1995, pp. 262–263). The cultural trends to which Herman (1995) referred included the disruption of traditional family and community ties, a greater emphasis on the patriarchal nuclear family, an increased pressure to satisfy the emotional needs of children and adults after the Second World War, and a loss of self in large corporations and institutions during postwar economic growth.

There was also gender disparity in the popularization of psychological theory, especially in relation to obesity. In the postwar USA, the desire to control weight manifested differently along gender lines. Dieting and weight management was predominantly directed toward (middle-class) women, and the psychosomatic explanation of emotional eating complemented the traditional belief that the constitution of a woman was innately weak due to the perils of the female life cycle. The early nineteenth-century "psychology of the ovaries" had established the prevalence of female hysteria and invalidism. The reinterpretation of hysteria in the second half of the nineteenth century as neurasthenia and neurosis by the mid-twentieth century entrenched the notion of female susceptibility to conditions stemming from emotional origins (Ehrenreich and English, 2005). The cultural tolerance for women's bodies was also narrowing in the postwar period. The emphasis on a secure domestic home life as the cornerstone for national stability was, in part, reflected in the ability of women to fulfill the roles of a capable homemaker, nurturing mother, and sexually attractive wife (May, 2008; Metzl, 2003; McLaren, 1999; Caplan and Feldstein, 1998; D'emilio & Freedman, 1988). The valorization of thinness to demonstrate self-control and domestic success intensified the need for women to reduce and manage their body weight (Stearns, 2002; Schwartz, 1986), and gave increased credence to the role of the expert in domestic life and diet culture (Ehrenreich and English, 2005).

Postwar mental health professionals encouraged people to view psychology as an acceptable way to cope with the challenges of the modern lifestyles and popular literature providing the conduit inundating mainstream America with popularized psychological theories. Newspaper and magazine articles now addressed the topic of psychology, providing a new language to discuss emotions and normalizing psychological theory by relating it to experiences in everyday living. Major national newspapers published reports related to the usability of psychiatry in all areas of postwar living (Folliard, 1946; Menninger, 1946; Browning, 1946, 1953). Women's magazines were also influential in raising popular consciousness around understanding the psyche (Moskowitz, 2001, pp. 167–172). The common categories of articles relating to mental health included voyeuristic pieces that revealed the emotional problems of other women and psychological self-help features with titles such as "What Sends People to Reno?" (Bender, 1948), "Are You an Everyday Neurotic?" (Zolotow, 1957), "What's Your Emotional Breaking Point" (Colley, 1955), and "Who's Happy and Why" (Brothers, 1961). In addition, regular advice columns gave practical guidance from a psychological perspective such as the long-running "Making Marriage Work" by psychologist Clifford R. Adams in *Ladies' Home Journal.*

The popularization of the psychoanalytic explanation for obesity in the late 1940s and 1950s recontextualized the theory of an oral fixation addiction to the public. The edification of medical research papers around obesity in popular literature was produced both by the researchers themselves as well as by editorial staff, and pieces were often syndicated to appear in truncated form in daily newspapers (Smith, 1987). In order to give scientific legitimacy and a tenuous link to the medical research on which the popular articles based their relevance or cultural authority, health experts (often physicians or psychiatrists) were employed in the articles to comment on the psychology of obesity and provide weight control advice to the audience. Bruch was a prolific writer both in academic publications and of popular articles and was often called upon as an expert commentator on obesity and weight loss solutions. Bruch was astute in minimizing the vulgarization of her research, but even her self-authored pieces conformed to the structure, tone, and language of the popular literature of the period (Bruch, 1949, 1954a, 1954b, 1955). The emotional eating explanation was also embraced by other journalists and advice columnists, many of whom gained notoriety as lay weight loss experts in the popular press, such as, Ida Kain, William Laurence, and Antoinette Donnelly.

Popular articles from the 1950s tended to be based on a pattern that emphasized the problem of obesity and framed the oral fixation theory as a medical breakthrough (Smith, 1987). The articles that focused on problem-solving stressed the growing challenge of obesity in terms of both the health and social aspects, and heralded the new psychological theory for obesity as a valuable medical advance. The explanation-orientated articles placed emphasis on the usability of the "discovered" medical theory by first discrediting previous medical beliefs to identify a gap in the knowledge so that the reader then anticipated an explanation. In a 1950s article "Obesity," published in *Good Housekeeping*, the glandular and hereditary theories were cursorily debunked, and the author pointed out that it is not physiology that was to blame but rather emotional tension: "The person who has a deep, if hidden, sense of not being loved, not being wanted, often satisfies his need for love by eating" (Davis, 1950, p.13). In most cases, the popular pieces that outlined the dangers of obesity and the psychological dimension to overeating gave vague advice on how to address the emotional conflict reverting back to prescribed diet plans. In these instances, the trivialization of the process to lose weight often gave the impression that weight control was straightforward and was within the control of the individual. The message emphasized was that weight loss could be achieved by exercising self-control around food and taking a cheerful outlook on life, which corresponded to the established moralistic dieting ideals that would have been familiar to an American audience.

The translation of the psychology of obesity, in order to make it easily palatable to a mainstream audience, vulgarized the medical rhetoric. In general, this was seen in the omission of any discussion around psychoanalytic addiction theory. Instead, a simplified psychosomatic connection was accentuated between emotional maladjustment or disturbances (possibly being based in childhood experiences but which could also be derived from traumatic lifestyle events such as a divorce) and overeating as a means to soothe the list of emotions mentioned in the article, namely unhappiness, anxiety, nervousness, worry, and frustration. For example, a report published in *The New York Times* on the psychology of obesity in 1950 summarized the theory in a typically simplistic manner:

> The newest reason put forward by some members of the medical profession, is that we allow our emotions to get away from us and think ourselves into fatness. The idea is that when something is wrong psychologically we may try – unwillingly – to seek compensation through food, beyond our natural demands.
>
> (Whalen, 1950, p. SM12)

This process tended to remove orthodox Freudian language and minimize any sexual drive or intrapersonal theories such as oral fixations, the oedipal complex, and autoplastic materialization.

Rather, the use of stereotypes to create a relatable emotional eating identity to mainstream America, along with the inclusion of a less formal tone and the use of non-technical terms, were the common features of popularized literature surrounding obesity. The commonly used description which stereotyped the emotional eater was that of a person (often female) who looked to shift the blame of excess fat away from her behavior. Instead, another reason was given: a hereditary condition or a glandular imbalance. This person also underestimated the volume of food they consumed, offering excuses that they "eat like birds" or "live off a diet of coffee" (Davis, 1950). According to popular literature, it was their difficulty dealing with emotional problems that resulted in the overeater using food to cope with stressful experiences.

Lay expert weight management

The 1940s psychological understanding of obesity was not just popularized and disseminated to mainstream America through media outlets; the ideas were also actively absorbed and adapted by laypeople into eclectic weight management programs. One of the most widespread popular responses to the increase in attention to obesity and the reconceptualization of overeating as a psychological problem was the postwar group weight loss movement. From 1948, weight loss groups emerged throughout North America with names such as *Take Off Pounds Sensibly*, *Fatties Anonymous*, *Calories Anonymous*, *Overeaters Anonymous*, *Weight*

Watchers, and *Diet Workshop*. These groups were founded on the notion that over-eating was due to psychological maladjustment and that the psyche of the person had to also be addressed if weight was to be effectively managed. These weight loss groups developed programs based on group therapy and the program of *Alcoholics Anonymous* (AA) (Parr, 2014, pp. 774–776). How the mind–body connection was conceptualized and translated into specific group practices depended on the interpretation of the specific lay community regarding the exact nature of the psychological problem. The lay understanding of health and illness of these postwar weight loss groups was not static, and shifted in parallel with medical science, which resulted in changes to group practices and structure (Parr, 2014, pp. 778–788). But it was the flexibility presented in the translations by lay communities of the psychology of obesity that allowed for eclecticism, adaptation, and commercialization.

One of the earliest and most popular weight loss groups was *Take Off Pounds Sensibly*, commonly referred to by the acronym TOPS. The organization was founded in 1948 by Esther Manz, a 40-year-old housewife from Milwaukee, Wisconsin. In a similar manner to other postwar groups, the style developed by TOPS was built on the "lay expert" understanding of obesity. By 1950, the popularized psychological understanding of obesity as oral fixation was dominant in American culture, as was the idea that the psychological approach of releasing traumatic emotions would help address the problem of obesity (Parr and Rasmussen, 2012). The founding members of TOPS believed that excess weight was due to using food to address feelings of loneliness, despair, and unhappiness. To manage body weight effectively, the individual had to build personal fortitude to cope with emotional distress without resorting to food as a solace. The practices developed by TOPS reflected this basic ideology of the group: that overeating was due to emotional distress that was within the individual's power to control and manage (Manz, 1956). The TOPS program used three interrelated approaches to help members manage their weight, including play psychology, competitions based around weight loss, and popularized AA customs. The combination of these methods constituted the foundation of the TOPS program.

It was important to the founding members that TOPS applied a playful element to the serious and highly stigmatized task of weight management. The play psychology adopted by TOPS was understood to address the neurosis and accompanying anxiety that the fat person was believed to experience by allowing self-expression and the cathartic release of repressed emotions in a safe environment. The spirited and often childlike activities were genuinely intended to combat the stigma of obesity and reflected the psychoanalytic influence in approaching weight management. In a Freudian sense, this widespread use of play psychology was aimed at encouraging regression to assist the personality to dissolve and reorganize, to allow the ego to mature past the oral stage of development and heal past psychological injuries (Parr and Rasmussen, 2012). Arguably, the dominance of play-inspired practices, initiated by founding members of TOPS, was a central way in which the popularized psychology of the 1940s was applied; painful emotions and traumatic experiences, that were understood to be the cause of obesity, were best approached in a playful, humorous, and fun manner within a supportive group environment. Such practices included a theatrical weigh-in ritual, playful chapter names and slogans, sing-a-longs, and parlor games (Parr, 2014). The founding methodology of TOPS, based on dominant psychiatric ideas of the late 1940s, constructed an enduring organizational framework for the group that has survived to the present day, and it was mimicked to various degrees by later postwar weight loss groups.

Conclusion

The idea of eating to relieve emotional tension was one of the most popularized narratives, and continues to be included in discussions around obesity today. In this chapter I have argued that this popular representation had its roots in the 1940s psychiatric understanding of obesity that presented the reason we overeat as being due to unresolved psychological conflict originating in childhood. According to mid-twentieth-century psychiatry, food became associated with love and was used by fat individuals as a compensation for dysfunctional parental affection as well as a defense mechanism against further rejection.

Throughout the 1950s these ideas were popularized and propagated by American culture to categorize the emotional eater as a person who temporarily eased unhappy emotions with food. The successful translation of the psychosomatic ideas concerning the cause of obesity outside professional medicine may be explained, in part, by the practical psychoanalytical approach characterized by Bruch that eased the popularization process. It may also be understood within the confluence of complementing postwar trends that helped galvanize the psychological basis for overeating, especially to the predominantly female audience that was the target of the burgeoning weight loss industry. Most notably, it was the period that saw the emergence of a group approach for weight loss that absorbed and assimilated popular ideas concerning obesity and weight loss to develop practices, based on the psychological model of obesity, for a rapidly growing dieting culture.

A layer of complexity was added to the emotional eating metaphor with the rise of behavioral theories for obesity. The popularized emotional eating concept was expanded, and now, rather than overeating being solely due to internal conflict, one could also overeat in response to external stress such as a demanding boss or arguments with a spouse. Behavioral psychology also supplied specific, non-technical actions which people could adopt at home to manage the environment that was the "trigger" of overeating. The pragmatism of behaviorist theory lent itself to popular culture and to lay expert weight loss communities where it was intermingled with surviving psychoanalytic ideas.

Since the 1950s, studies surrounding obesity have been contested across a number of disciplines which have developed increasingly more complicated and technologically driven theories to explain why we get fat. Psychologists, psychiatrists, sociologists, physicians, and researchers in the life sciences have all published studies on the reason people become obese and have contended for professional authority to direct medical treatment and shape public health policy. These explanations of obesity negotiate the intersection between biology, psychology, and the environment, as well as the role individual agency plays in lifestyle conditions. The psychoanalytic theory for obesity has been rejected by medical research, but the metaphors of emotional eating continue to hold resonance in mainstream culture. Returning to the popular example of *The Biggest Loser*, Ali Vincent, the first female to win the USA competition in 2008, recounted in her biography the "emotional void" she had been filling with excess food (Vincent, 2009). The audience learned of Vincent's troubled childhood and turbulent family relations (especially with her mother) throughout the season of the show and this was a major attribute interwoven into her weight loss story (*The Biggest Loser*, Smith *et al.*, 2008).

The longevity of the theory of emotional eating in popular culture may be understood not only in terms of the established cultural dimension to obesity, but also in the wider shifts in the approach to health care in the second half of the twentieth century. The fat body has an extensive history of being associated with undesirable traits related to race, class, and behavior. Nineteenth- and twentieth-century representations of the primitive "other"," or a social group that impinged upon societal norms from suffragists to capitalists, have often been depicted in the fat body as a visual symbol of denigration, immorality, or gluttony (Farrell, 2011). More recent understandings of the fat body have also reinforced patriarchal gender dynamics, with the emotional eating model resonating with the nineteenth-century notion of female invalidism due to nervous disorders.

In popular culture, obesity was viewed not merely as a physical handicap or a mental illness, but instead has occupied an ambiguous position between the two classifications, sharing elements from both but with the main defining feature being that the fat body was entirely within the control of the individual. This moralistic emphasis on willpower and individual responsibility supported the biopsychosocial model of chronic disease after the Second World War. As Porter has argued, health care "developed a model of prevention that primarily focused on changing individual behavior rather than addressing the social structural determinants of health and disease" (Porter, 2006, p. e399). There has recently been a shift toward recognizing and regulating the contributing environmental factors in obesity. Yet, popular discourse continues to use the metaphor of emotional eating. The enduring nature of this idea reinforces social stigmas and continues to endorse a construction of the self that values the belief that the fat body can be understood and regulated through a mind–body framework.

Notes

1 In this chapter, the term *psychosomatic* is defined as a physical condition that is initiated or exacerbated by psychological factors (APA, 1980). It is acknowledged that the primary cause of obesity is a positive energy balance within the body. However, the

explanation for the energy imbalance has, since the 1940s, involved a psychological dimension. The definition of "psychosomatic" in relation to obesity has changed across the second half of the twentieth century, with the explanation of the psychological factors shifting from intrapersonal conflict (APA, 1952) to emphasize the relationship of the individual with environmental stimuli (APA, 1980).

2 There are a large number of magazine articles, blogs, and self-help books that discuss emotional eating (too many to list here). A selection of recent examples include Kelly, n.d.; Emotional Eating, 2016; Alexandra, n.d.; Kromberg, 2013; Dryja, 2014; Roth, 2003; Gould, 2007; McKenna, 2014.

References

Alexandra, Z. (n.d). The #1 cause of emotional eating & weight gain: Stress. *Eating Like A Goddess Blog*. Available at www.eatlikeagoddess.com/articles/the-1-cause-of-emotional-eating-weight-gain-emotional-stress/.

American Psychiatric Association. (1952). *Diagnostic and Statistical Manual of Mental Disorders, First Edition*. Washington, DC: APA.

American Psychiatric Association. (1980). *Diagnostic and Statistical Manual of Mental Disorders, Third Edition*. Washington, DC: APA.

Bender, J. (1948). What sends people to Reno?. *Ladies' Home Journal*, April, p. 268.

British Broadcasting Corporation. (2015). *What's the Right Diet For You*. Available at www.bbc.co.uk/programmes/p02ddsd9.

Brothers, J. (1961). Who's happy and why. *Good Housekeeping*, May, p. 28.

Browning, N.L. (1946). Psychology of the sexes is need. *Chicago Daily Tribune*, September 22, p. C8.

Browning, N.L. (1953). We're not losing our minds. *Chicago Daily Tribune*, October 4, p. D19.

Bruch, H. (1939a). The Fröhlich syndrome: Report of the original case. *American Journal of Diseases of Children, 58*(6), 1282–1289. Available at http://archpedi.jamanetwork.com/.

Bruch, H. (1939b). Obesity in childhood: I, Physical growth and development of obese children. *American Journal of Diseases of Children*, *58*(3), 457–484. Available at http://archpedi.jamanetwork.com/.

Bruch, H. (1939c). Obesity in childhood: II, Basal metabolism and serum cholesterol of obese children. *American Journal of Diseases of Children*, *58*(5), 1001–1022. Available at http://archpedi.jamanetwork.com/.

Bruch, H. (1940a). Obesity in childhood: III, Physiologic and psychologic aspects of the food intake of obese children. *American Journal of Diseases of Children*, *59*(4), 739–781. Available at http://archpedi.jamanetwork.com/.

Bruch, H. (1940b). Obesity in childhood: IV. Energy expenditure of obese children. *American Journal of Diseases of Children*, *60*(5), 1082–1109. Available at http://archpedi.jamanetwork.com/.

Bruch, H. (1941). Obesity in childhood and personality development. *American Journal of Orthopsychiatry*, *11*(3), 467–474. Available at http://archpedi.jamanetwork.com/.

Bruch, H. (1943). Psychiatric aspects of obesity in children. *American Journal of Psychiatry*, *99*(5), 752–757. Available at http://archpedi.jamanetwork.com/.

Bruch, H. (1948). Psychological aspects of obesity. *Bulletin of the New York Academy of Medicine*, *24*(2), 73–86. Available at www.ncbi.nlm.nih.gov/pmc/articles/PMC1871113/.

Bruch, H. 1949). Overweight children. *Good Housekeeping*, March, p. 86.

Bruch, H. (1954a). Why do people eat too much. *Mademoiselle,* June, p. 55.

Bruch, H. (1954b). When not to diet. *Colliers*, February 5, p. 82.

Bruch, H. (1957). *The Importance of Overweight*. New York: W.W. Norton & Company.

Bruch, H. and Touraine, G. (1940). Obesity in childhood: V. The family frame of obese children. *Psychosomatic Medicine*, 2(2), 141–206. Available at http://archpedi.jamanet work.com/.

Burdon, A. and Louis, P. (1951). Obesity: A review of the literature, stressing the psychosomatic approach. *The Psychiatric Quarterly*, 25, 568–558.

Bychowski, G. (1950). On neurotic obesity. *The Psychoanalytic Review* (1913–1957), 37, 318–319.

Caplan, P. and Feldstein, R. (1998). Mother blaming. In M. Ladd-Taylor and L. Umansky, *"Bad" Mothers: The Politics of Blame in Twentieth-century America*. New York: New York University Press.

Colley, D. (1955). What's your emotional breaking point?. *Cosmopolitan*, February, p. 12.

Danowski, T. and Winkler, A. (1944). Obesity as a clinical problem. *The American Journal of the Medical Sciences*, 208(5), 622–630.

Davis, M. (1950). Obesity. *Good Housekeeping*, May, p. 13.

Dawes, L. (2014). *Childhood Obesity in America*. Cambridge, MA: Harvard University Press.

D'emilio, J. and Freedman, E.B. (1988). *Intimate Matters: A History of Sexuality in America*. Chicago, IL: University of Chicago Press.

Dryja, A. (2014, October 5). Try these powerful tools To stop emotional eating. *MindBody-Green Blog*. Available at www.mindbodygreen.com/0-15554/try-these-powerful-tools-to-stop-emotional-eating.html.

Dwyer, J.T., Feldman, J.J., and Mayer, J. (1970). The social psychology of dieting. *Journal of Health and Social Behavior*, 269–287. Available at www.jstor.org/stable/2948575?origin=JSTOR-pdf.

Ehrenreich, B. and English, D. (2005). *For Her Own Good: Two Centuries of the Experts' Advice to Women*. New York: Anchor Books.

Emotional Eating. (2016). *Women's Health and Fitness Magazine*. Available at www.womens healthandfitness.com.au/diet-nutrition/healthy-eating/278-emotional-eating.

Farrell, A.E. (2011). *Fat Shame: Stigma and the Fat Body in American Culture*. New York: New York University Press.

Folliard, E. (1946). Battlefield psychiatry can smooth the peace: "Morale" the goal. *The Washington Post*, June 23, p. B1.

Goldblatt, P.B., Moore, M.E., and Stunkard, A.J. (1965). Social factors in obesity. *Jama*, 192(12), 1039–1044. Available at http://jama.ama-assn.org/.

Gould, R. (2007). *Shrink Yourself: Break Free From Emotional Eating Forever*. Englewood Cliffs: Wiley.

Hale Jr., N.G. (1995). *The Rise and Crisis of Psychoanalysis in the United States: Freud and the Americans, 1917–1985*. Oxford: Oxford University Press.

Hamburger, W.W. (1951). Emotional aspects of obesity. *Medical Clinics of North America*, 483–492.

Herman, E. (1995). *The Romance of American Psychology. Political Culture in the Age of Experts*. Berkeley: University of California Press.

Ikin, S. (2016, February 18). Emotional eating fuelling Australia's obesity epidemic. Australian Broadcasting Corporation. Available at www.abc.net.au/news/2016-02-18/emotional-eating-fuelling-australias-obesity-epidemic/7175204.

Kaplan, H. I., Kaplan, H. S., and Leder, H. L. (1957). The psychosomatic management of obesity. *New York State Journal of Medicine*, *57*(17), 2815–2826.

Kelly, A. (n.d.). Stop emotional eating. *Shape*. Available at www.shape.com/healthy-eating/diet-tips/stop-emotional-eating.

Kromberg, J. (2013). Emotional eating? 5 reasons you can't stop. *Psychology Today Blog*, September 18. Available at www.psychologytoday.com/blog/inside-out/201309/emotional-eating-5-reasons-you-can-t-stop.

Levy, D. (1941). Maternal overprotection. *Psychiatry*, *4*(4), 567–626.

Manz, E. (1956). *How to Take off Pounds Sensibly: A Guide to Health and Happiness*. Milwaukee, WI: TOPS Inc.

May, E. T. (2008). *Homeward Bound: American Families in the Cold War Era*. New York: Basic Books.

McKenna, P. (2014). *Freedom from Emotional Eating*. New York: Hay House.

McLaren, A. (1999). *Twentieth-century Sexuality: A History*. Englewood Cliffs, NJ: Wiley-Blackwell.

Menninger, W. (1946). The promise of psychiatry. *The New York Times*, September 15, p. SM6.

Metzl, J. (2003). *Prozac on the Couch: Prescribing Gender in the Era of Wonder Drugs*. Durham, NC: Duke University Press.

Moore, M. E., Stunkard, A., and Srole, L. (1962). Obesity, social class, and mental illness. *Jama*, *181*(11), 962–966. Available at http://jama.ama-assn.org/.

Moskowitz, E. S. (2001). *In Therapy We Trust: America's Obsession with Self-fulfillment*. Baltimore, MD: Johns Hopkins University Press.

Newburgh, L. (1931). The cause of obesity. *Journal of the American Medical Association*, *97*(23), 1659–1663. Available at http://jama.jamanetwork.com/.

Newburgh, L. (1942). Obesity. *Archives of Internal Medicine, 70*(6), 1033–1096. Available at http://archinte.jamanetwork.com/.

Parr, J. (2014). Obesity and the emergence of mutual aid groups for weight loss in the post-war United States. *Social History of Medicine*, *27*(4), 774–776, hku020.

Parr, J. and Rasmussen, N. (2012). Making addicts of the fat: Obesity, psychiatry and the "fatties anonymous" model of self-help weight loss in the post-war United States. *Critical Perspectives on Addiction (Series Volume 14)*, 181–200.

Penick, S. B., Filion, R., Fox, S., and Stunkard, A. J. (1971). Behavior modification in the treatment of obesity. *Psychosomatic Medicine*, *33*(1), 49–56.

Porter, D. (2006). How did social medicine evolve, and where is it heading? *PLoS Medicine*, *3*(10), e399. Available at http://dx.doi.org/10.1371/journal.pmed.0030399.

Rascovsky, A., Rascovsky, M. W., and Schlossbery, T. (1950). Basic psychic structures of the obese. *The International Journal of Psycho-Analysis*, *31*, 144–149.

Rasmussen, N. (2012). Weight stigma, addiction, science, and the medication of fatness in mid-twentieth century America. *Sociology of Health and Illness*, *34* (6), 880–895.

Rasmussen, N. (2015). Stigma and the addiction paradigm for obesity: Lessons from 1950s America. *Addiction*, *110*(2), 217–225.

Reeve, G. H. (1942). Psychological factors in obesity. *American Journal of Orthopsychiatry*, *12*(4), 674–678.

Richardson, H. B. (1946). Obesity as a manifestation of neurosis. *The Medical Clinics of North America*, *30*, 1187–1202.

Roth, G. (2003). *Breaking Free From Emotional Eating*. New York: Plume.

Schick, A. (1947). Psychosomatic aspects of obesity. *The Psychoanalytic Review (1913–1957)*, *34*, 173.

Schwartz, H. (1986). *Never Satisfied: A Cultural History of Diets, Fantasies, and Fat.* New York: Free Press.

Smith, D. E. (1987). The process of popularization — Rewriting medical research papers for the layman: Discussion paper. *Journal of the Royal Society of Medicine, 80*(10), 634.

Smith, T., Jones, M., and Brown, C. (2008). *The Biggest Loser.* Available at www.nbc.com/the-biggest-loser.

Stearns, P. N. (2002). *Fat History: Bodies and Beauty in the Modern West.* New York: New York University Press.

Stunkard, A. and Levitz, L. (1974). Effective elements of behavior modification: Results from a large-scale study of treatment for obesity. *Journal of Psychiatric Research, 10*(2), 162.

Vincent, A. (2009). *Believe It, Be It: How Being the Biggest Loser Won Me Back My Life.* Philadelphia, PA: Rodale Books.

Whalen, R. (1950). We think ourselves into fatness. *The New York Times*, December 3, p. SM12.

Zolotow, M. (1947). Are you an everyday neurotic? *Cosmopolitan*, April, p. 39.

5 Impossible illnesses

Decolonizing psychosomatic medicine

Amba J. Sepie

The phenomenon of the psychosomatic illness, spectral, yet apparent, and unclear in its causation, resists easy classification. The "realness" of an illness that cannot, or will not, be "properly" situated within the biomedical paradigm attracts both questions and doubts. *It is all in her mind* has been whispered since at least the dawning of psychiatry, although this was already well beyond the abandonment of the original traditions of those who would be called Moderns. Descartes' legacy, as extended and built upon by legions of scholars, is the dictum that things "of the mind" must remain "of the mind," and those of the body, contained. Within this chapter, I query how the designation of psychosomatic is situated with respect to this legacy, located as it is between the fixed categories of body and mind. What is also questioned is whether it is possible for this category of psychosomatic to exist at all, given that particular metaphysical inheritances have led, ideologically, to the practices of biomedicine within what we might call "the West." If, as is argued, the idea of the psychosomatic does not exist in the sense to which we are accustomed, then perhaps there are other sociocultural frameworks that can be invoked to rethink ideas about cause, symptom, illnesses, and healing.

The project of decolonizing medicine, to which this chapter is inherently linked, takes into account the displacement of other traditions of healing through the globalization of biomedicine, and attempts to address the assertions of neutrality and universality that have been made in its name. Decolonization, in general, refers to any project that critically assesses practices and discursive constructions that may be called culturally "Western," and interrogates their value for a given community. The decolonization of medicine, therefore, is engaged with the radical re-visioning of the body's relations with the environment, other people, and the terms by which bodily processes have been cross-culturally understood. Decolonization is important because a common assumption, deriving from a history of colonization and development discourses, is that non-Western peoples are "better off" with biomedicine, and for some complaints this is no doubt correct. However, I argue that biomedical practitioners and institutions cannot deal with all manner of complaints, but can only ever *partially* attend to the spectrum of human health-related phenomena, which renders them particularly ineffective when it comes to the illnesses that are categorized as psychosomatic.

Projects of this nature must take account of history, which, for medicine, involves the trajectory adopted by modern philosophical and scientific thought, an endeavor that divided mind and body more conclusively than even Descartes may have imagined. Elizabeth Grosz (1994, p. 1), who determines the Cartesian split to be the most influential philosophical legacy for defining knowledge, describes the body as a "blind spot," conceived of in terms of the mind–body split, but also a number of additional dualities:

> [M]ind and body, thought and extension, reason and passion, psychology and biology . . . sense and sensibility, outside and inside, self and other, depth and surface, reality and appearance, mechanism and vitalism, transcendence and immanence, temporality and spatiality . . . form and matter, and so on . . . [defining] the body in nonhistorical, naturalistic, organicist, passive, inert terms.

Modern medical practices are ultimately defined in accordance with such binaries. Deborah R. Gordon (1988), who examines the "Western" in Western medical practices, argues that there is some validity in referring to a consistent set of traditions we can call both Western and medical, albeit distributed to different degrees across time and space. Her view is that these Western medical practices, or *biomedicine*, carry certain assumptions which are both tenacious, and embodied in practices, while also operating as *background* assumptions, by which she means flexible, undefined, and taken-for-granted assumptions that are not typically questioned and may, therefore, be somewhat invisible informants of worldview (pp. 22–23). She writes: "we may increasingly speak of a social scientific/historical gaze turned on medicine, describing hidden cultural scaffolding and social processes that shape practice and knowledge" (p. 20).

Psychosomatic complaints occupy a shadowy place in this dual system, and are often precarious subject positions, classified poorly somewhere between the sharply defined edges of biomedicine and the liminal zones of religion, madness, and imagination. According to the Cartesian worldview, "the body is construed to work according to mechanical principles independent of the will, spirituality, and purposes of the subject . . . [this] orients biomedicine and provides its principal justification . . . and authority" (Schneirov and Geczik, 2003, p. 42). However, biomedical legitimacy extended to psychosomatic complaints may be difficult to achieve. The lived experiences of suffering from unacknowledged, or partially acknowledged, symptoms is impeded by the standardization of categories of empirical *data*, which insist upon the tracing of symptoms to particular kinds of causes, in accordance with the industrial model of the medicalized human being.

This issue of data and the related questions regarding validity were articulated best in 1973 by feminist philosopher Mary Daly, who bemoaned the processes by which marginalized ideas and knowledge(s) were purified by the prescriptions on scholarship and thought. Her insight is that:

> [T]he tyranny of methodolatry hinders new discoveries. It prevents us from raising questions never asked before and from being illumined by ideas that

do not fit into pre-established boxes and forms. The worshippers of Method have an effective way of handling data that does not fit into the Respectable Categories of Questions and Answers. They simply classify it as nondata, thereby rendering it invisible.

(Daly, 1985, p. 11)

Data, in academic terms, refers to information that will be counted as knowledge, and this is linked to an epistemological judgment about *fact status*, and a parallel axiological judgment about *value*. Data will be counted as data, or will not, in accordance with the degree of conformity it has with already established categories, which vary from one discipline or professional field to another.

Psychosomatic, therefore, is a label that is used to collate certain types of lived human experiences which appear to have similarities, and yet are classified as non-data in biomedical terms. This label can act to exclude these from the processes of being taken seriously as legitimate biological symptoms, with *causes*. Illness has to have data to be *real*. Symptoms have to be *symptoms of*.... However, psychosomatic illness has no data; it is a classification that names and reduces a lived experience, so that it may be contained within biomedical understandings of the body. As Laurence J. Kirmayer writes, "psychosomatic disorders have been incorporated into biomedicine as a class of not quite legitimate illnesses best handled by mental health practitioners" (1988, p. 64). Wherein the practice and study of psychosomatic medicine presupposes the concept of mind–brain relations, and is dependent upon the concept of classic symptomatic and comparative-objective diagnosis to remain an empirically respected science, it is generally only somatic phenomena that are admissible within the naturalistic paradigm.

It may be argued that *psychosomatic* is a status designation of a condition *similar* to illness which possesses elements of unreality, or invisibility; however, there is a sleight of hand in this process of naming which remains unexamined. First, the categorization of a condition as psychosomatic defines an illness as partially unreal, as based on the absence of a verified cause, or the lack of a quantitatively derived explanation. Second, having contained the experience with a definition of this kind, the new status of the complaint (imagined, or all in one's head) shifts the responsibility for taking it seriously from the biomedical practitioners to the head doctors – the psychologists and psychiatrists – and, either tacitly or overtly, to family, friends, priests, and rabbis. In this manner, the looping effect of referral between these two different sections of the biomedical professional world may result in individuals desperately seeking the recognition of their pain or symptoms in real, organic, and recognizable terms, rather than accept the stigmatization of a mental health diagnosis. Thus we must ask: to what extent is this paradigm and the different types of legitimacy that are granted, or withheld, by practitioners therein actually equipped to serve a healing or curative function for the person in question?

The psychosomatic is technically a sub-specialty of psychiatry – the symptoms are defined as *psychiatric*, and psychiatry itself is designated as a part of biomedicine (Ackerman and DiMartini, 2015). However, psychiatrists do not claim to deal expressly with causes, and do not claim to be involved in the treatment of medical,

biochemical, and physical diseases that can be "cured," although they may speculate on genetic and neurological origins. *Cure* is not a term used within psychiatry,
which puts the psychiatric patient in a difficult position (Schioldann and Berrios,
2015). By locating the illness "in the head" the *patient becomes morally responsi-*
ble for causing the condition in a manner that does not apply so readily to physical
causes (Kirmayer, 1988, p. 75). Furthermore, the patient typically loses a degree
of social status as a rational and agential individual when submitting to psychiatric treatment. As Kirmayer notes, Cartesian dualism has dictated that mind and
body are typically split into voluntary and intentional (mental), and involuntary
and accidental (bodily) – "real" sickness in Western terms just "happens" to us –
"a person cannot be 'really' sick until an autonomous biological process takes
hold" (p. 75). Such a diagnosis "transforms the real into the imaginary . . . [and]
psychosomatic diagnosis creates the reality it intends to describe . . . [forging] a
link between mind, as subject, and body as object" (p. 65).

The process of naming, using this *particular* term within this particular paradigm, moves the lived experience from the real complaints that biomedical practitioners can "see" to the category of conditions that cannot be "seen," or that have
questionable ontological status. Ontological categories are just that, however;
prescriptions for the conditions of reality which appear to be concrete when, in
fact, they are the products of decisions regarding what ought, and ought not, to be
permitted to exist. Ontology, in turn, is based on cosmological predicates. All reli-
gions and belief systems have charter myths (or origin stories) which set up these
ontological categories of being – angels, demons, nature Gods – that are based
on stories about creation. These origin stories establish the *cosmology*. The story
of science added new creation stories to the old Judeo-Christian stories, which
had the effect of replacing the Garden of Eden with the Big Bang, and Heaven
with material death. This generated a new salvation story predicated on avoidance
of death at all costs and – critically – *while remaining tied* to Judeo-Christian
concepts of morality, progress, and purpose. This fusion of science and religion
has set a cosmological framework that determines what can and cannot be "real"
(the ontological criteria). Just as gods, ghosts, diviners, prophets, and animistic
beliefs are excluded from the set of approved entities, so too are explanations for
illness that do not conform to the established rules by which we are obligated to
understand the human being. This dominant cosmology does not routinely allow
invisible entities, nor illnesses without visible causes, since these are ontologically impossible according to a naturalistic cosmology.

The deception, then, is that the name itself (i.e. psychosomatic) is an invented
classificatory device that no more belongs to the biomedical paradigm than the set
of complaints to which it refers. By designation of the overarching cosmological
predicates, *it is ontologically impossible for any "real" condition to be psychoso-*
matic. An illness has to be transformed into either a mental or a physical issue, to
be classed as psychosomatic – it cannot be both as the cosmology does not allow
for this. Psychosomatic illnesses cannot be entertained from the perspective of the
worldview which has spawned the biomedical paradigm – there can be no such
category according to this worldview.

It is the *classification* of psychosomatic, therefore, that is the actual unreal entity (or ontological impossibility), existing only to fulfill the criteria designated by the cosmological predicates for biomedical classification, values, knowledge legitimacy, and practices, as set down and then expanded upon via the scientific worldview. Psychosomatic, as a biomedical diagnosis, shifts some of the harder problems of mind–body consciousness temporarily out of the realm of science and into psychiatry, which, as stated earlier, promises no cures. To make a lived experience *real* within this paradigm can only be achieved by either the "crossing-over" of the experiencing person into a diagnosable category (finally finding a cause, location, or source that was previously obscured); or, via the promised progress in biomedicine (based on new discoveries in genetics, the neurosciences, or other technological advances) which alters the status of the complaint sufficiently for it to be recognized as ontologically real.

A disclaimer is needed here, lest it be assumed that this is some sort of conspiratorial action on the part of physicians or researchers. To the contrary: the paradigm is faithfully reproduced, by the actions of its adherents, to achieve exactly what it has been set up to do. However, it is not equipped to deal with the entanglements of body and mind as intimated by the idea of mind–body, when the paradigm itself deems that these should be kept separate. Mind–body cannot be included in the dataset, as *there is no such permissible biomedical combination*. Once the psychosomatic label has been attached to a lived experience, any questions asked by a medical practitioner (who is thus internal to the biomedical framework) ultimately query whether the illness phenomenon a person is experiencing is "real," and there is only one possible answer – it is not – because the label designated the answer as a priori non-data. Psychosomatic, in biomedical terms, has become a euphemism for symptoms that are imaginary and fictional – *mythos*, not logos.

The invisibility status that is generally attached to psychosomatic illness may be constructed as something resembling a fiction, yet ironically it is one that cannot be visually or conceptually well represented in the very media which handle fiction. One of the only reference points within popular culture seems to be the attachment of mental instability to images of deviance. Theories of deviance hold that deviant categories are "clustered" together, so difficult or antisocial characteristics or behaviors create cross-labelling: the label of psychosomatic can "trigger" cross-labeling to mental illness, which is regarded as deviant (see O'Neill and Seal, 2012). In daily life, popular culture, and general media, such clusters are reproduced in a manner that sequesters persons labeled as deviant and metaphorically confines them to liminal spaces such as prisons, hospitals, asylums, nightclubs, drug dens, and so forth.

According to Lawrence Rubin (2012, p. 288), pop culture "sells" with depictions of deviance: insanity, wounded heroes, wicked women, and criminality in all its forms:

> post-traumatic stress disorder, post-partum depression, sociopathy, and psychosis – powerful words that can and do influence the very manner in which

we look upon and attempt to make sense of others. . . . What are we to do with the haunting image of the sociopathic killer, the suffering military veteran, the deranged psychotic lesbian or pathetic stutterer? How easily and casually do we compartmentalize?

These are gross caricatures that inscribe difference and encourage fear in equal measure: deviance clusters that are examples of consequence. Such images serve as an explicit warning should one's *own* mind not "stay put" and remain obedient.

Culpable in the perpetuation of such stereotypes are theological concepts of divine punishment, sin, and guilt, which underpin a great number of modern Westernized societies. As the Judeo-Christian Bible warns, madness is the result of disobedience. "Moses warns his people that if they 'will not obey the voice of the Lord your God or be careful to do all his commandments and his statutes . . . the Lord will smite [them] with madness and blindness and confusion of mind' (Deut 28:15, 28)" (Harper, 2009, p. 2). This theological pronouncement is not at all obsolete but informs modern secular life through the inherited metaphysical scaffolds that have been directly absorbed into our social norms and institutions.

The concept of *governmentality*, as proposed by Michel Foucault, seems particularly relevant to this within societies that are characterized by mechanisms of social control, wherein citizens remain bound to ideas of obedience (Foucault *et al.*, 1991). Tacit and explicit compliance with a number of social conventions, such as obedience to authority figures (judges, doctors, parents, teachers), or prescriptions enforced institutionally, may be a strategy for avoiding the consequences (both secular and divine) that may manifest upon the individual. However, as Eliot Freidson (1975) notes, the physician, while a professional, may not always be an authority when it comes to best practices for dealing with complex – including psychosomatic – complaints. In the absence of a satisfactory treatment option, responses that are thought to lack rigor but are *in-paradigm* (such as psychiatry) may be acceptable, even when these are lacking a clear scientific foundation. Freidson notes that medical practitioners are "obliged" to orient "toward intervention irrespective of the existence of available knowledge. The practitioner is more comfortable doing something . . . [being] inclined to fear doing nothing – and so is led to use drugs and other procedures more than might be indicated by academic (and scientific) standards" (1975, p. 163).

Popular television culture depicts modern medical heroes dealing with "real" issues in a high-tech, high-pressure surgical environment, rushing in to the emergency rooms with last-minute revelations, saving lives, and warding off death. This "recovery narrative," as argued by Johanna Shapiro, is very straightforward: "patient gets sick; patient receives medical intervention; patient recovers and returns to pre-illness life" (2011, p. 69). These stories tend toward neat classifications of bodies and patients (identical, warehoused, numbered, machine-like) and hero-doctors. Popular culture can set up the expectations of *real medical students* and *real patients* who enter the *real hospitals* expecting to be heroes and extras in the quintessential story of How We Beat Death since our recent rescue from the plague, smallpox, and tuberculosis: all of which are clearly just a breath away from returning should medicine ultimately fail. In this way, just as we "make" popular culture, popular culture representations also help shape modern societies. When a small child says, "I want to be a doctor," it is safe to assume that they are drawing upon romanticized notions of what doctors actually do, and some of this derives from an overarching faith in medicine: on the screens, and in our homes. As Gordon states, "medicine offers a strong sense that humans can overcome nature, no longer a victim, but in the omnipotent driver's seat" (1988, p. 41). She writes that naturalism and biomedicine free human beings from the supernatural; elevating us from the weaknesses of the body through the presentation of an ideal of absolute freedom: "beyond the ravages of time – beyond death" (pp. 23–40).

Joseph Turow and Rachel Gans-Boriskin (2007, p. 280), in their survey of 50 years of doctors on television, suggest that formulaic depictions of medical practices present

> health care dilemmas within the traditional formula's rather tight focus on doctors in a hospital setting . . . characters rarely point out that the problems they confront have significance far beyond their particular hospital . . . nurses, social workers, and other members of the health care team hardly exist . . . patients and their friends and relatives appear to have little impact on health care decisions.

Television has always emphasized the role of the physician and the power of medicine. Although doctors have become a little more like "real people" over time (for instance, they can fall sick, die, fail, or be put at risk) their position as hero is sustained by the depictions of their struggle to be good and ethical, all while remaining problematically *mortal*.

The oddly theological or Olympian quality afforded to these representations of hero-doctors is difficult to resist: following Gordon's insight, it is entrancing to consider and invest in the dramatic play of heroic salvation set against the tyrannical persistence of mortality. Popular culture further normalizes the reverence, awe, and authority granted to biomedicine, given the persistent and subtle reminders of the chaos that would surely ensue in its absence. Gordon writes that even as advancing biomedical technologies *continually* fail to subvert mortality, or to raise us above being "merely human," the quest for it persists (1988, pp. 40–42). Pointing out the paradox, she asks: does this not put us squarely "back in the supernatural camp which science aspired to leave?" (p. 40).

Medical-scientific and industrial advancement is sanctioned at the expense of other worldviews, and other alternatives to mainstream thinking about health. For instance, the rule for handling the phenomenon of chronic pain requires an injury or illness which can be correlated to the experience of pain in order for it to be real, *despite* evidence, witness, and testimony as to the existence of suffering. Elaine Scarry (1985), in a brilliant discussion of how other people's experiences become visible or invisible to us, argues that both material and immaterial "objects" are pressed in and out of existence according to the relations between categories of objects, and according to complex agendas. She writes that pain events happening within a person's physical body "may seem to have the remote character of some subterranean fact, belonging to an invisible geography that, however portentous, has no reality because it has not yet manifested itself on the visible surface of the earth" (p. 3).

Pain is not always biomedically visible. Pain does not always have *data*, so there is a question as to where it should be "attached": to the physical body, the brain, the mind, or the imagination. As Jean E. Jackson argues, chronic pain, when designated as "no longer biologically useful," serves an illegitimate function and is, itself, illegitimate (1992, p. 140). Pain is an invisible entity, with no place in the ontological register. Scarry's prose is evocative here:

> Vaguely alarming, yet unreal, laden with consequence yet evaporating before the mind because not available to sensory confirmation, unseeable classes of objects such as subterranean plates, Seyfert galaxies, and the pains occurring in other people's bodies flicker before the mind, then disappear.
>
> (Scarry, 1985, p. 4)

Pain, when constituted as a medical problem, tends to be fragmented into a series of dichotomies which map onto the cultural logic of biomedicine, resulting in the conclusion that pain experiences are entirely individual rather than inter-subjective (Kleinman *et al.*, 1992, pp. 8–9). Naturalistic assumptions demand, ultimately, reductionism to objective observance of biological mechanisms. Gerard P. Montague explains that:

> In a naturalistic paradigm, we would expect that all of our conscious states or experiences could at least in theory be shown to correlate in some way with some physically detectable neuronal (or other) activity in some part of the body – primarily in the brain.
>
> (2012, p. 154)

These are facts, these are *data*. A brain is a visible thing, the first cause that is identical with the mind, and the center of human experience and expression. From the perspective of medical science, the brain is the modern location of what used to be called God. The brain (as concept) co-opts a person's agency: the brain is in charge, the brain acts, does, determines; it is the designated source of everything a human being is; the agreed-upon site of consciousness, and of the Western modern self.

Lay conceptions, or public understandings of medical science and scientific processes, as covered extensively in the work of Brian Wynne (Irwin and Wynne, 1996; Wynne, 2006), tend toward unstable ideas of science that are tremendously elevated, poorly defined, and often incorrect. Such positions tend toward the acceptance of the idea that everything "lives" in this brain – imagination, reason, madness, religion, deviance, passion, intellect, intuition – instructions for the gross mechanical actions of the physical body, and instructions for the unconscious workings of the inner cogs which keep the heart pumping and the lungs breathing. Furthermore, it is not that there is *no* cause for those mysteries, illness or otherwise, that remain unexplained; rather, it is acceptable to think that there *must not yet be a sufficient understanding* of the causes. The entire project of scientific inquiry hangs on the same logical projection: that it is simply a matter of time. Pharmacology, genetic research, and the neurosciences promise the psychological equivalent of mortgage securities to the medically disenfranchised.

Whatever biomedical definitions, practices, objects, or promises are employed, the nature of humankind (according to naturalism) originates with one rather narrow slice of European thinkers, whose philosophical scaffolds and sureties have come to engulf the world through the mechanisms of, first, colonialism, and, second, globalization. Consider, for example, the strong sense of durability conjured up by the following. According to medical historians the origins of psychosomatic, as both a term and a concept, can be *retrospectively* applied: for instance, the figuring of illness as an imbalance of humors in Hippocratic thought, the diseases of passion in Galen, and the writings of Maimonides in the twelfth century (see Lipowski, 1984). This appears plausible: if medical historians can find it in the past, then must not this framing have existed then, as it does now? Alas, no. To project ideas that could now be called psychosomatic onto precursory worldviews, such as found in Greece, or in Maimonides, *constructs* the validity of the use of the term by conveying the appearance of fact, truth, and surety throughout time, as if there is, indeed, something called psychosomatic that existed *prior* to the creation of the concept itself, when, in fact, there was not. To the contrary, there were a *number* of different cultural contexts for understanding the nature of human health and sickness, incorporating different models of the human body.

Generations of scholars, writers, and practitioners working in this field have long labored with a choice between two equally unpleasant alternatives – to accept the brain–mind–body distinctions and reside within the paradigm, or to reject it and risk marginalization equal to that of their patients. This quandary fueled the invention of psychiatry in the early nineteenth century and psychology toward its close: how to legitimately practice a science of the mind *without* substantive curative measures for mental complaints, on the basis of a particular view of the human body and brain. Those who locate themselves within the field are therefore faced with questions of credibility which cannot be easily resolved. Direct engagement with the lived experiences that are labeled as psychosomatic ultimately *contradicts* established scientific-cosmological notions regarding human bodies, illnesses, and the nature of humankind. As such, there have emerged, over time, a number of specialists who exist on a spectrum in terms of how they mediate, integrate, or ignore the dual concepts of mind and body. Of these, the philosophical tenets of traditional and indigenous healing practices have become increasingly popular under such headings as mind–body medicine, bio-psycho-social approaches, eco-psychology, quantum medicine, and related modalities that incorporate a broader, holistic, or *ecological* view of the human being.

In medical anthropology also, ethnographers have long been "testing spirituality on their own pulses" (Turner, 2006), engaging with diverse worldviews in order to learn and understand the applications of successful healing modalities within other cultural complexes. Cultural perspectives, under the heading of *ethnomedicine*, may retain alternative cosmological notions that map illness, health, body, mind, and spirit in different ways. These perspectives teach that the body is the *most* subjective site for the appearance of disharmony and sickness, not the least. Bodies may also be thought of quite differently. Ning Yu's work on the Chinese heart is a good example of different conceptualizations of the human body that demonstrate distinct ideas about biology and cause (Maalej and Yu, 2011; Yu, 2009). Traditional Chinese thought encompasses physical, social, and spiritual well-being as interrelated, and uses a model of the body quite unlike the one generated out of the context of Cartesian dualism.

In such examples, the human is considered in relation to other people, other species, and the wider environment, and all of this is potentially a source for what is elsewhere called a psychosomatic illness. The human body is but one site in a series of interlinked human–environment relationships that can be destabilized, and the sources of disharmony can extend to the multispecies kin group, to other species, to events in ancestral history, or to other features of lived daily reality which are not considered causative within a biomedical paradigm. The Māori view of self, for instance, may include land as a part of the *actual body* of the self, as kin that is not separate from personhood: geographical features are agential in the co-construction of health and well-being (Mark and Lyons, 2010, p. 1760). Trespassing against land, when it is intrinsically thought to carry notions of personhood, is sufficient to destabilize the health of an individual, their kin group, and the natural or multispecies community that surrounds them.

Such ideas are found widely distributed across diverse traditional and indigenous contexts, with substantive similarities in how disharmony is then mediated and corrected by traditional healing practices. Consider the concept of *territory*, for example. Juan Echeverri (2005, pp. 234–235), who describes this in the context of the Colombian Amazon, notes that *first territory* may be thought of as the mother's body: her womb, and then her breasts. Throughout the lifespan of a person, the range is extended; first to other, shared, territories in the natural environment, wherein nourishment derives, and then to the bodies of other humans with whom partnership is sought. Thus the territory is "naturalized" through this idea of body, producing a relational fabric which extends beyond the individual. This is how relationship with place may be thought of in symbolic terms as an extension of the self. Similarly, the instability of the idea of human "species-membership" among shamanistic practitioners in diverse Amazonian and Siberian cultural complexes incorporates an integrated view of human-animal-nature that defies classification, disrupting "rational" rules of nature–culture separateness (Goulet and Miller, 2007; Harris and Robb, 2012; Vilaça, 2005).

Even complaints that arise from injury in such contexts have a *relational* component, which means they have significance or layered *meanings* that are situated according to a network of relationships. There are no "accidents" in most ethnomedical contexts. Health concerns are significant, taken seriously, and respected as manifestations of imbalance that must be mitigated; not only for the individual, but also for the health of the whole group, the surrounding environment, and in order to maintain good ecological relations. Traditional Chinese thought, despite great modifications and increased urbanization, still incorporates powerful ideas about kinship, responsibility, and awareness of place that can impact the health of an individual. Collective responsibilities, reciprocity in all relationships, respect, and care for all manifestations of life on earth are the central tenets of any fundamental ethical position internal to indigenous, traditional, and holistic worldviews: in other words, we are all properly responsible for one another.

Such a notion stands in radical opposition to the individualistic and atomistic concepts of the body with which we are familiar, and requires a different understanding of cause and effect. This is a *fundamentally different* view of the human: one that has synergy with ecologically oriented systems thinking (wherein relationships replace subject–object relations), and is philosophically compatible with holistic psychotherapeutic practices. One such practitioner, Brian Broom, states that in some cases, "the emergence of an illness in a culture may be less a function of what actual historical life-experiences the individual has had, and more a representation of the spiritual state of that culture" (2007, p. 201). The loss of community and the rise of individualism within modern, urban, capitalistic, atomized societies is a disease burden in and of itself, affecting relations within and between individuals who struggle to harmonize with their designated roles, and who are increasingly alienated from both their habitat and other humans. This is supported by the increasing speculation that the rise in mental illness diagnoses (such as depression and anxiety) among modern urban peoples is intrinsically linked to the type of societies in which we live.

Gay Bradshaw suggests that the miscomprehension that modern Westernized individuals have about the world is, overwhelmingly, that we are all disconnected, or in some way separate from nature when, in fact, such a divide is illusory (2013, p. 134). The great revelation in this idea is the possibility that if we are *not* actually disconnected, perhaps the societies we co-construct reflect the *quality* of our connections, or lack thereof. Her insight shows a thoughtful application of traditional and indigenous ways of thinking about human–environment relationships to illustrate the degree to which we are embedded in, and affected by, such relationships, whether we realize this or not. These are important observations for the decolonization of medicine and human–environment relations as a whole.

Although they are not yet fully encompassing this idea, holistic psychotherapeutic approaches do focus upon the individual as *socially* embedded, sufficiently so as to manifest physical symptoms that are responses to relationships with other people. Using the idea of *somatic metaphor*, Brian Broom (2007, p. 88) argues:

> The popularly held crude distinction between real physical diseases with no "psychosomatic" element, and those often reversible illnesses that are "psychosomatic" is grossly inadequate . . . somatic metaphors compel people to reflect on what a "person" (with or without disease) actually is, to reflect on our fundamental nature. How can a meaning, a subjective idea, have a highly specific metaphorically physical outcome in the body that is conventionally seen as a sort of machine? . . . we have, in the somatic metaphor, a major challenge to such materialist assumptions. I see somatic metaphors every day. If we see them, it is a duty to point out their implications.

Somaticization, the process to which Broom refers, is defined by Siegfried Zepf (2014, p. 36) as:

> a perspective from which a somatic disease is conceived as a specific strategy in which psychic conflicts have found a pathological solution. The somatic diseases are conceived as elements which meaningfully complete an individual life history and whose significance is no longer transparent to the subject.

Broom's work is focused upon the meanings embodied by humans within their concepts of self, body, and experience. Broom also has dual qualifications of immunologist and psychotherapist, and has gradually appropriated the insights of psychotherapy to assist in dealing with conditions that were unresponsive to conventional immunological treatments (detailed in Broom, 1997, 2007). He gives a number of examples describing how somatic metaphors manifest. One example is of a child who manifested the symptoms of her mother's undisclosed rape experience (Broom, 2007, pp. 163–168). While this would not be considered at all unusual within ethnomedicine wherein cross-generational or cross-species transfer of symptoms is acceptable, the metaphysical predicates for biomedicine would not readily admit this sort of account as data. To complicate the matter further, the situation was resolved following the *mother's* therapy, not the child's – an impossible resolution. Holistic approaches such as this anchor the illness in a "network of intersubjective interweavings and places the historically developed specificity of a person at its centre" (Zepf, 2014, p. 38). In other words, the human is relational – the patterns and interconnections described by Zepf and Broom simply relay, in the language of psychotherapy, the observations made by traditional and indigenous healers.

Broom also questions why we should automatically assume that the relationship between experience and disease is an individual matter:

> In the West we have emphasized individuality, and the separateness of bodies, to the point that we can hardly imagine disease as arising from disordered

relationships, let alone as an expression of someone else's experience. What we forget is that our individuality is really a semi-stable reality, very subject to change, and it often takes much energy to achieve and maintain.

(Broom, 2007, pp. 163–164)

A practitioner who can interpret the environmentally situated human body as a site of interactions, information, and emotional exchange may be well equipped to dismantle experiences of illness by making visible the causes that biomedical practitioners cannot see.

In conclusion, it would appear that ethnomedical and holistic psychotherapeutic perspectives can offer good answers to difficult questions. For those who live with psychosomatic diagnoses, the approaches considered here represent opportunity; the chance for their illnesses to become visible, independent of the constructed apparatuses of a biomedical approach (and its mediatized representations) that can neither contain, nor comprehend, their particular afflictions. With regard to the wider project of decolonizing medicine, it is hoped that this chapter may provide encouragement to look more deeply into the cosmological constructions that influence how truths are established and power is maintained. The impacts of colonization are intensely personal, as evidenced by the representations, ideas, and philosophies that are foundational to the establishment of biomedicine and the categorization of the modern, Western self as somehow elevated and separated from the natural world. Decolonization queries the acceptance of the cosmological predicates upon which modern societies, and a wealth of social interactions, are now based.

There is no more radical agenda than to suggest cosmological change, nor one that attracts more resistance, than to break with what Bradshaw calls the "concept and agenda" defining Western society, that which fragmented the world "into brittle edges and wounded psyches by humanity's contraction into the bare bones of survival" (Bradshaw, 2013, p. 133). The reduction of what are termed psychosomatic complaints to the two poles of body and mind are, at root, an outcome of a particular cosmology which is, plainly put, a set of ideas, agreed upon and reproduced across systems of thought and practice, although not the only ones from which we might choose.

References

Ackerman, K. and DiMartini, A. F. (eds). (2015). *Psychosomatic Medicine*. New York: Oxford University Press.

Bradshaw, G. A. (2013). Living out of our minds. In P. H. Kahn Jr. and P. H. Hasbach (eds), *The Rediscovery of the Wild* (pp. 119–139). London: MIT Press.

Broom, B. (1997). *Somatic Illness and the Patient's Other Story*. London; New York: Free Association Books.

Broom, B. (2007). *Meaning-full Disease: How Personal Experience and Meanings Cause and Maintain Physical Illness*. London: Karnac.

Daly, M. (1985). *Beyond God the Father: Toward a Philosophy of Women's Liberation*. Boston, MA: Beacon Press.

Echeverri, J. Á. (2005). Territory as body and territory as nature: Intercultural dialogue? In A. Surrallés and P. García Hierro (eds), *The Land Within: Indigenous Territory and the Perception of the Environment* (pp. 230–246). Copenhagen: IWGIA.

Foucault, M., Burchell, G., Gordon, C., and Miller, P. (1991). *The Foucault Effect: Studies in Governmentality*. Chicago, IL: University of Chicago Press.

Freidson, E. (1975). *Profession of Medicine: A Study of the Sociology of Applied Knowledge*. New York: Dodd, Mead.

Gordon, D. R. (1988). Tenacious assumptions in Western medicine. In M. M. Lock and D. R. Gordon (eds), *Biomedicine Examined* (pp. 19–56). Dordrecht; Boston: Kluwer Academic.

Goulet, J-G., and Miller, B. G. (eds). (2007). *Extraordinary Anthropology: Transformations in the Field*. Lincoln: University of Nebraska Press.

Grosz, E. A. (1994). *Volatile Bodies: Toward a Corporeal Feminism*. Bloomington: Indiana University Press.

Harper, S. (2009). *Madness, Power and the Media: Class, Gender and Race in Popular Representations of Mental Distress*. London; New York: Palgrave Macmillan.

Harris, O. J. T. and Robb, J. (2012). Multiple ontologies and the problem of the body in history. *American Anthropologist, 114*(4), 668–679.

Irwin, A. and Wynne, B. (1996). *Misunderstanding Science? The Public Reconstruction of Science and Technology*. Cambridge; New York: Cambridge University Press.

Jackson, J. E. (1992). "After a while no one believes you": Real and unreal pain. In A. Kleinman, P. E. Brodwin, B. J. Good, and M-J. D. Good (eds), *Pain as Human Experience: An Anthropological Perspective* (pp. 138–168). Berkeley: University of California Press.

Kirmayer, L. J. (1988). Mind and body as metaphors: Hidden values in biomedicine. In M. M. Lock and D. R. Gordon (eds), *Biomedicine Examined* (pp. 57–93). Dordrecht; Boston: Kluwer Academic.

Kleinman, A., Brodwin, P. E., Good, B. J., and Good, M-J. D. (1992). Pain as human experience. In A. Kleinman, P. E. Brodwin, B. J. Good, and M-J. D. Good (eds), *Pain as Human Experience: An Anthropological Perspective* (pp. 1–28). Berkeley: University of California Press.

Lipowski, Z. J. (1984). What does the word "psychosomatic" really mean? A historical and semantic inquiry. *Psychosomatic Medicine, 46*(2), 153–171.

Maalej, Z. A. and Yu, N. (eds). (2011). *Embodiment Via Body Parts: Studies from Various Languages and Cultures*. Amsterdam: John Benjamins.

Mark, G. T. and Lyons, A. C. (2010). Maori healers' views on wellbeing: The importance of mind, body, spirit, family and land. *Social Science and Medicine, 70*(11), 1756–1764.

Montague, G. P. (2012). *Who Am I? Who Is She? A Naturalistic, Holistic, Somatic Approach to Personal Identity*. Heusenstamm: Walter De Gruyter.

O'Neill, M. and Seal, L. (2012). *Transgressive Imaginations: Crime, Deviance and Culture*. Basingstoke: Palgrave Macmillan.

Rubin, L. C. (2012). Introduction and Afterword. In L. C. Rubin (ed.), *Mental Illness in Popular Media: Essays on the Representation of Disorders* (pp. 5–8; 288–289). London; Jefferson: McFarland.

Scarry, E. (1985). *The Body in Pain: The Making and Unmaking of the World*. New York: Oxford University Press.

Schioldann, J. and Berrios, G. (2015). "The meaning of the symptom in psychiatry. An overview" by Hans W. Gruhle (1913). *History of Psychiatry, 26*(2), 214–232.

Schneirov, M. and Geczik, J.D. (2003). *A Diagnosis for Our Times: Alternative Health, from Lifeworld to Politics*. Albany: State University Press of New York.

Shapiro, J. (2011). Illness narratives: Reliability, authenticity and the empathic witness. *Medical Humanities, 37*(2), 68–72.

Turner, E.L.B. (2006). Advances in the study of spirit experience: Drawing together many threads. *Anthropology of Consciousness, 17*(2), 33–61.

Turow, J. and Gans-Boriskin, R. (2007). From expert in action to existential angst. In L.J. Reagan, N. Tomes, and P.A. Treichler (eds), *Medicine's Moving Pictures: Medicine, Health, and Bodies in American Film and Television* (pp. 263–281). New York: University of Rochester Press.

Vilaça, A. (2005). Chronically unstable bodies: Reflections on Amazonian corporalities. *The Journal of the Royal Anthropological Institute, 11*(3), 445–464.

Wynne, B. (2006). Public engagement as a means of restoring public trust in science – Hitting the notes, but missing the music? *Community Genetics, 9*(3), 211–220.

Yu, N. (2009). *The Chinese Heart in a Cognitive Perspective: Culture, Body, and Language*. Berlin: Mouton de Gruyter.

Zepf, S. (2014). Thoughts about psychosomatic symptom formation. *The Scandinavian Psychoanalytic Review, 37*(1), 36–47.

6 Narrative coherence and medical explanations of psychosomatic pain

Seamus L. Barker and G. Lorimer Moseley

Introduction: Narratives and medical explanations of pain

"Psychosomatic pain" is not only described, but also routinely explained, in personal accounts of pain sufferers, in popular culture, and in medical discourses. When personal accounts of pain come from white Western populations they commonly take on a narrative form, drawing upon various metaphors, even while incorporating causative explanations of the pain aiming at medical or scientific legitimacy (see e.g. Good *et al.*, 1994). Such accounts commonly emphasize an "organic" cause of "real" pain, positioned in dichotomous opposition to "psychosomatic" explanations burdened with implications that the pain is imagined or otherwise unreal. In popular culture, explanations of illness and disease similarly draw upon metaphors that facilitate a dualistic division, such that the symptomatic body is represented as either having been invaded or threatened by an external enemy, or else afflicted by the mind of the sufferer themselves (see e.g. Sontag, 1991). In this sense, such accounts from popular culture – whether in public political discourses, news reportage on health, the Internet, or self-help books – typically depend on narrative elements as they strive for explanatory coherence. Medical explanations, meanwhile, are obliged to be objective, rational, scientific, though, like narratives, also coherent. In this chapter, we will investigate whether the medical classifications of "Psychogenic Pain Disorder," "Somatoform Pain Disorder," "Pain Disorder," and "Somatic Symptom Disorder" – as they appear in various editions of the *Diagnostic and Statistical Manual* (*DSM*), published by the American Psychiatric Association (APA) – in fact rely on structures and features found in popular culture narratives, as those psychiatric classifications also strive for explanatory coherence.

"Psychosomatic pain" is defined by *Mosby's Medical Dictionary* as "pain that is caused in part by psychologic factors" (O'Toole, 2013, p. 1485). What similarities or differences exist between the ways in which such causes and effects are handled in popular cultural narratives on the one hand and in technical medical explanations on the other? Ricoeur suggests that narrative is constituted by the retrospective positing of causal and meaningful connections between disparate events, a process he calls "emplotment" (Dowling, 2011, pp. 9–17). Comparably, Thagard notes that attempts to account for causation in medicine necessarily

begin from observing correlation between certain events (including the development of a disease), and proceed to the retrospective search for causal connections
among them (1998, p. 66). Just as Ricoeur suggests that narrative is constituted
by coherence, achieved through "emplotment" (Dowling, 2011, p. 5), so does
Thagard note that "the justification of scientific theories including their postula-
tion of theoretical entities is a matter of explanatory coherence, in which a theory
is accepted because it provides a better explanation of the evidence" (1998, p. 70).
Notably, though, Thagard cautions: "medical explanation is not just story telling,
since a good medical explanation should point to all the interacting factors for
which there is causal evidence and for which there is evidence of relevance to the
case at hand" (1998, p. 74).

It seems, however, that there is a potential for *narrative* coherence – rather than
strictly scientific coherence – to shape a medical explanation. Karhausen notes
that, in attempting to explain disease causation, various dubious assumptions are
commonly made, in particular that a single explanatory factor can be identified;
that causes are never chain-like; that, in the case of chronic disease, the causes are
"continuant" or ongoing (Karhausen, 2000, pp. 62–63). These common assumptions are at odds with what Hucklenbroich calls "the real organization of processes
in biological systems" which he considers to be constituted by "cyclical, feed-back,
self-referential, and self-processing network[s] of structures and processes" that
furthermore are "polyvalent, changing, and ambivalent concerning their causal . . .
meaning" (2014, pp. 610–611). Pain, too, is often understood to arise from a
complex biological system (see e.g. Moseley, 2013) – with multiple, interacting,
causally circular features – a model that might threaten the *narrative* coherence of
any attempted explanation. Indeed, the common tendencies noted by Karhausen,
while dubious from a scientific or philosophy of science perspective, may all be
understood to enhance *narrative* coherence by facilitating a movement toward *closure* and explanatory simplicity, these latter which, in narrative terms, we could
call *minimalism* or *reduction*. Carroll (2007) suggests that narrative closure "tran-
spires when all of the questions that have been saliently posed by the narrative get
answered" (p. 4), and it may be suggested that the achievement of such a moment is
surely also a key objective of medical explanation. In working toward explanatory
closure, the aforementioned common assumption that Karhausen identifies – that
a singular or constant explanatory factor or *causal agent* exists – may be related to
a *narrative* tendency to impute causal responsibility to a single, indivisible entity,
such as a character. This idea will be developed below.

Causal entities, narrative *actants*, and explanatory coherence

Various theorists of narrative (beginning with Aristotle) have noted that narratives generally present events that are implicitly or explicitly *causally connected*
through emplotment, while also suggesting that plot and character in narrative
are mutually constitutive (Abbott, 2008, p. 42). In literary studies, structuralist
narratologists identified basic functions performed by characters that were shared

across the range of narratives they analyzed, as they sought to understand the common mechanics of plot function. Greimas (1983) used the term *actants* to denote not only characters but also non-human, nominalized entities that were causes of effects, or the sites of effects – such as *The United States*, *The Black Dog* (of depression), or *Cancer*. *Actants* – as nouns that typically enact verb functions (or receive transitive verb functions) – play a central role in sustaining a sense of causal connection in narrative (Mel'čuk, 2015, p. 227), potentiating emplotment and coherence. Regarding disease, Thagard suggests that, as well as functioning probabilistically, causal explanations are strengthened by the incorporation of a biological mechanism to link cause and effect (1998, p. 66). Thagard defines a mechanism as "a system of parts that operate or interact like those of a machine, transmitting forces, motions, and energy to one another" (1998, p. 66). Thagard's idea of mechanism shares some similarities with the structuralist narratologists' concepts of the relationship of *actants* to plot. Dowling summarizes Greimas's work in this field thus:

> Greimas's system begins from the notion of *actant*: not an actual character, but the formal function that any character may fulfill in a narrative structure . . . Greimas's first move is to isolate six *actantial* categories: A desires B . . . an act of communication relates A to B . . . or there is a pragmatic relation between A and B.
>
> (Greimas, 2011, p. 42)

We see, then, that just as one part of a mechanism can act on another part – for example, imbuing kinetic or heat energy, thus transforming it – so does one *actant* act upon another: imbuing "pragmatic," that is, material, change; attracting, or being attracted to, another *actant* through the operation of "desire"; altering another *actant*'s potential, or state, through an act of "communication" (Dowling, 2011, p. 42). Thagard notes that, as well as identifying mechanisms, physicians and epidemiologists, in "finding correlations and eliminating alternative causes," are, in effect, inferring the existence of "theoretical *entities*" that function as "causal powers" (1998, p. 66; emphasis added). Regarding explanations of "psychosomatic pain," we will shortly see that entities with causal powers, or their mechanisms, can be made to function similarly to *actants* in narratives. As we proceed, we will bear in mind the question of whether the use in explanations of something like *actants* helps achieve explanatory coherency and closure, but also whether such usage comes at a price – perhaps of biological accuracy, inferential reasoning, or sensible clinical responses. If such a price must be paid to use *actants* to structure explanations, is there also a simultaneous potential for these structures to be manipulated to generate rhetorical power and persuasive effects?

Another narratologist, Brémond (1973), distinguished between *agents* – as *causes* of effects – and *sufferers* – those that suffered the consequences (that is, they *received* effects). Propp (1968) identified a role he labeled the *helper*, that functioned to aid the hero in folklore, as well as the converse, the *opponent*. We will draw eclectically upon this felicitous nomenclature, to illustrate the ways in which implicitly narrative structures are commonly used to enhance – or impose – explanatory coherence. That is, when analyzing various accounts of psychosomatic pain – whether from popular culture or technical medical explanation – we will, where pertinent, identify a *sufferer* (of pain), a *causal agent* (of the pain), a *helper* (the diagnosing doctor who names the *causal agent*), and, occasionally, an *opponent*. The utility of this approach will become clear in practice.

Disease entities, diagnosis, and responsibility

Hucklenbroich, working on the history and theory of medicine, suggests that "disease entity" is the central notion undergirding medical pathology (2014, p. 609). The concept of "disease entity" takes diseases to be "natural classes," "analogous to the conceptual structures of plant and animal in biology" (Hucklenbroich, 2014, p. 611). Hucklenbroich goes on to specify the principles on which the idea of "disease entity" are based – "completeness" and "unambiguousness" (2014, pp. 613–614). Hucklenbroich resists any sense of disease "gradualism" that would suggest a shading of degrees between health and illness, or between person and disease (2014, p. 627). Anything pathological must be "an instance of [at least] one disease entity" (Hucklenbroich, 2014, p. 613). Any pathological conditions that are not part of a disease entity "do not exist in reality" (Hucklenbroich, 2014, p. 613). The principles of the concept "disease entity," then, are those of *closure*, as they demand a rigid and totalizing judgment of inclusion/exclusion. On this view, diseases, as instances of disease entities, are, like persons (or plants or animals), defined by a clear boundary, unitary and indivisible, either complete and unambiguous – a thing-in-the-world – or not existing. Hucklenbroich further notes that the concept of "disease entity" covers not just signs and symptoms but, "particularly, the causal structure 'lying behind them'" (2014, p. 616).

Inseparable from the idea of "disease entity" is the idea of "diagnosis." Michael Bury's qualitative sociological research with sufferers of chronic illness draws out some of the important moral implications of interactions between issues of cause and diagnosis:

> Access to medical knowledge, at least in the case of physical illness, offers an opportunity to conceptualize the disease as separate from the individual's self . . . the separation of disease from self is a powerful cultural resource. The objectivity of disease provides, through medical science, a socially legitimate basis both for deviant behavior and clinical intervention. . . . To be able to hold the disease "at a distance", as it were, assists the claim that one is a victim of external forces. To do anything less is to accept fully the burden of responsibility.
>
> (Bury, 1982, p. 173)

Bury makes clear, then, the connection between a sense of *causal* and of *moral* "responsibility" in their relation to disease. The etymology of "diagnosis," according to the *Oxford English Dictionary* (2016), is from the Greek, *dia* (asunder) and *gignōskein* (perceive . . . to know), into *diagignōskein* (distinguish, discern), into Modern Latin and "diagnosis." To *know asunder* implies that what is discerned is that which is essentially divided from – other than – the body of the sufferer. It must be the doctor (narratively, the *helper*) who through the act of diagnosis not only names the disease entity (*causal agent*) but in so doing marks its division from the *sufferer*, absolving them of such "responsibility" in what we might call a cardinal moment of closure (Bury, 1982, p. 173).

It seems that an implicit *actant* structure that allocates moral, as well as causal, responsibility is embedded in dualistic ideas about disease. Boorse (2004, p. 86) suggests that:

> The idea that serious diseases excuse conduct derives from the model of the relation of agents to their own physiology. Unfortunately the relation of agents to their own psychology is of a much more intimate kind. The puzzle about mental illness is that it seems to be an activity of the very seat of responsibility – the mind and character – and therefore to be beyond all hope of excuse. . . . It is persons, not personalities, who are held responsible for their actions, and one central element in the idea of a person is certainly consciousness.

For Boorse, then, "mental illness" does not exist, insofar as, in the vast majority of cases, he considers the *sufferer* responsible for their own state of suffering, and thus not worthy of "special treatment" or having any "valid excuse for normally criticizable behavior" (2004, p. 84). On this basis Boorse would presumably consider psychogenic disorders, as "caused" by the *sufferer* rather than by organic disease, to not constitute illnesses, and their consequences to be similarly inexcusable (2004, p. 87). Suzanne O'Sullivan, a neurologist, wrote a book on psychosomatic disorders for popular consumption: *It's All in Your Head: True Stories of Imaginary Illness* (2015). For O'Sullivan, as for Hucklenbroich and for Boorse, the *causal agent* should normally be "the disease" – which is "organic" – and refers to "pathological disorders of the body, as opposed to disorders of the mind" (2015, p. 21). For O'Sullivan, where there is "no disease" the symptoms must be due to "psychological or behavioral reasons" (2015, p. 7). Reading these accounts coming from medical specialists and philosophers and historians of medicine, it seems that "disease entities," – construed as "natural classes" – and diseases – reified as "things" in the body – form the basis of diagnosis and of individual medical explanations. The indivisibility and boundedness of these constructs can be readily transposed onto the *sufferer*, as in O'Sullivan's explanation. That is, following the exclusionary *either/or* causal logic of dualism and the diagnostic principle of *closure*, if no disease can be found then the ill person becomes the singular agent, in narrative terms the *actant*, responsible – causally and morally – for their own suffering.

Within this dualist paradigm, when it comes to pain the *causal agent* or "disease entity" held responsible in medical explanations is generally an "organic lesion." *Mosby's Medical Dictionary* defines "lesion" as a "wound, injury, or pathologic change in body tissue" (O'Toole, 2013, p. 1025). Such terms encapsulate both cause and effect, implying external circumstance acting upon the body – the injury or disease entity from without, and the resultant lesion within – which, in a reductively dualistic framework, subsequently determines pain. Within this framework, the *sufferer* of pain is a passive recipient, free from implications of causal or moral responsibility.

The other side of this dualistic coin consists in illnesses not grounded in a known and detectable organic pathology: the "symptom-based diagnoses" of which Aronowitz writes (2004, p. 66). What is at stake if ongoing pain is under-stood to not be caused by an observable lesion or organic disease entity? A 2013 meta-synthesis of qualitative research into the experience of chronic low back pain reveals the common experience of stigmatization, which was linked spe-cifically to having "a lack of diagnosis" (Snelgrove and Liossi, 2013, p. 292). Subjects remained "determined to establish a legitimate cause" of their pain, but reported being "viewed as culpable," with the assumption that their "symptoms" were "all in the mind" (Snelgrove and Liossi, 2013, p. 292). We see, then, that to suffer from chronic pain but not have a diagnosis of a legitimated disease entity is to experience being judged by society. We see also the ease with which suffer-ers of pain can reproduce the very dualistic discourse that is implicated in their stigmatization, since it could be suggested that symptoms are always experienced subjectively, and are never strictly *in* the body. But what does it mean for a range of symptoms to be brought to closure under the signifier, "all in the mind"? And what work does this closure do for the coherence of medical and popular accounts of "psychosomatic pain"?

Psychogenic pain: the divided *sufferer* as *causal* agent

First let us consider the concept of "psychogenic" or "psychosomatic pain," which latter is defined by *Mosby's Medical Dictionary* as "pain that is caused in part by psychologic factors" (O'Toole, 2013, p. 1485) (even as contemporary neurobiological accounts suggest that pain is *always* caused in part by psycho-logic factors). In popular culture, self-help books have regularly incorporated the basic causal model found in *Mosby's*. The very title of Kenneth Pelletier's *Mind as Healer, Mind as Slayer: A Holistic Approach to Preventing Stress Disorders* (1977) suggests that the "Mind" can function precisely as either the *causal agent* ("Slayer"), or else, in narratological terms, the *helper* ("Healer"). Pelletier (1977, pp. 15–16) narrates:

> An individual is confronted with a stressful situation which is extremely dif-ficult for him . . . to resolve. . . . He makes an unconscious choice which allows him a means of coping with this irresolvable situation. . . . One means of reso-lution is to develop a psychosomatic disorder . . . which [leaves him] . . . inca-pacitated and released from the responsibilities which weigh . . . upon him.

O'Sullivan's book was published almost 40 years later. Therein she speculates whether a patient, disabled by a "psychosomatic disorder" six years ago, "might have chosen a wheelchair over a psychiatric diagnosis," although O'Sullivan believes that "if such a choice had ever been made, it had not been a conscious one" (2015, p. 53). Evident in both of these accounts is a strong overlap between narrative coherence and explanatory coherence in the movement toward closure. The narrative construction explains a psychosomatic disorder by assuming retro-spectively that because the symptoms of the disorder have certain consequences – avoidance of a stressful situation and release from certain responsibilities – then therefore the psychosomatic disorder and its symptoms must have developed *in order to* achieve those ends. This teleological logic is, according to Ricoeur, con-stitutive of narrative, since characters – and narrators – act to cause effects largely on the basis of their goals and purposes (Dowling, 2011, pp. 43–49). Also worth noting in their similarity are the implicit *actant* structures of the above passages. Here, the cause of the psychosomatic symptoms is made singular, indivisible, and very clearly arising from the activity of an *agent* – since a "decision" or "choice" must be made in order to become ill. Yet, in positing this process as occurring in the unconscious, the *causal agent* is, in an important way, divided from *the suf-ferer* and established, in terms of *actant* structure, as a double, or doppelganger. This accordingly allows the *sufferer* to be absolved of moral responsibility for their own transformation.

The two accounts differ in an important way. For Pelletier, it is precisely because doctors fail their patients in the moment of diagnosis – by using the signifier "psychosomatic" to signify not psychogenesis but rather that their illness "has no real basis" – that the doctor, instead of fulfilling the role of *helper*, has turned into an *opponent* – that *actant* that thwarts the mission of the protagonist – while concomitantly the role of *helper* can be fulfilled by the suf-ferer's "Mind" (Pelletier, 1977, p. 13). O'Sullivan focuses on the same moment, but instead suggests it is the failure of the *sufferer* to accept the appropriate – psychological – diagnosis that effects the transformation, as this failure becomes one and the same as their "choice" of a wheelchair and physically disabling symptoms. In O'Sullivan's version, then, the doctor remains a *helper*, but is thwarted by the *sufferer* who, in their "choice," becomes both *opponent* to the doctor/*helper*, and *causal agent* of their own suffering. We see, then, that a simple *actant* structure, and a teleological progression, together potentiate an implicit moral as well as causal accounting, apparently enhancing explanatory coherence and achieving closure via rhetorical, rather than necessarily scien-tific, elements.

What of the domain of medical explanation? "Psychogenic Pain Disorder" appears in the *Diagnostic and Statistical Manual* for the first time in its third edition (*DSM-III*), published in 1980. This condition is defined by "severe and prolonged pain" that is however "inconsistent with anatomic distribution of the nervous system" such that the pain "cannot be adequately accounted for by known pathology," or where "the complaint of pain is grossly in excess of what would be expected from the physical findings" (*DSM-III*: APA, 1980, p. 249). In addi-tion, "Psychological factors are judged to be etiologically involved in the pain" (*DSM-III*: APA, 1980, p. 249). "Psychogenic Pain Disorder" is clearly distinguished in *DSM-III* from "Malingering" in which, as a point of contradistinction, "the symptom production is under the individual's voluntary control" (*DSM-III*: APA, 1980, p. 248). "Psychogenic Pain Disorder" thus implicitly assumes an internal division in the mind of the sufferer, such that it is some unconscious part that fulfills the role of *causal agent*, as occurs in Pelletier's and O'Sullivan's explanations. Just as narrative logic dominates those accounts from popular culture, so too is it evident in the *DSM-III*, since the acceptable types of "evidence" of psychological etiology (causation) are all dependent on either the retrospective imputing of causal connections based on temporal sequence ("a temporal relationship between an environmental stimulus that is apparently related to a psychological conflict" and the onset of pain), or on teleology, such that outcomes ("support", "avoidance") are taken as the intended goals which the development of pain will achieve (*DSM-III*: APA, 1980, p. 249).

The power of implicit *actant* structure: the culpable *sufferer*

In the *Revised Third Edition – DSM-III-R* – published in 1987, "Psychogenic Pain Disorder" was abandoned in favor of "Somatoform Pain Disorder." In "Somatoform Pain Disorder" the essential feature is "preoccupation with pain for at least six months" (*DSM-III-R*: APA, 1987, p. 266). Beyond this criterion, whereas *DSM-III* insisted upon etiological psychological factors, the *DSM III-R* notes that they may be "evidence," or "no evidence," of psychological factors as etiological (1987, p. 265). Similarly, there may be evidence, or no evidence, of organic pathology (*DSM-III-R*: APA, 1987, p. 266). These criteria may seem inconsistent, and indeed we would suggest that what ultimately coheres them into an effect of closure is the establishment of a single, indivisible *actant* – the *sufferer* as *causal agent* – made to bear responsibility for the psychiatric disorder, as constituted through their agentic, not passive, pathological "preoccupation with pain" (*DSM-III-R*: APA, 1987, p. 266).

Significantly, what is common to these various accounts is an absence of any acknowledgment that medical knowledge may be limited. Such an acknowledgment would weaken the power of the doctor/*helper* to authoritatively make a diagnosis, and thus potentially, in this context, dispossess them of agency and reduce them to a non-character in the clinical drama. In *DSM-III's* account of "psychogenic pain," just as in O'Sullivan's clinical anecdote, when confronted with pain that "cannot be adequately accounted for by known pathology" the doctor's role as *helper* is still preserved, precisely by transforming the unaccountable symptoms into the psychiatric pathology of the *sufferer*: who can now be diagnosed as the *causal agent* (*DSM-III*: APA, 1980, p. 249). *DSM-III-R* similarly establishes something observable and knowable by the doctor – *preoccupation* – as the central criterion of a diagnosable psychopathology, although here there is no division of the mind to separate moral culpability from the *sufferer*.

Returning to popular culture, Ben Goldacre, a London-based doctor, wrote in the *British Medical Journal* about an angry letter that was sent to a radio station where he had spoken on air about risk factors and treatments for chronic back pain. The letter read:

> I would take issue with your speaker Ben Goldacre, who, if I recall correctly, said that 90% of back problems are psychosomatic disorders. What planet is he on? Whilst I would agree that there are a lot of schmucks out there that want to sit around and skive off work every day (and thereby make the problem even worse) . . . never tell me my backache of 20 years is imaginary. OKAY?
>
> (Goldacre, 2007, p. 801)

Here, a teleological sense is created, as "psychosomatic disorders" are associated with the goal of "skiving off work every day" (Goldacre, 2007, p. 801). Yet the writer seems to acknowledge that such "psychosomatic disorders" do not simply involve malingering, as he says that to "sit around" really will "make the problem even worse" (Goldacre, 2007, p. 801). Still, all of this seems to be "imaginary" when compared with the bodily reality of "my backache" (Goldacre, 2007, p. 801). In terms of causal effects, this account of "psychosomatic disorder" is confused and confusing, yet it retains a degree of narrative coherency and *closure* through its simple *actant* structure – in which the *sufferer* and the *causal agent* are made one. What is striking is that, for all its apparent incoherency, this account's structural operation – as supported by the cohering function of the signifier, "imaginary" pain – is ultimately relatively similar to that of *DSM-III-R*, although here the binding of moral to causal responsibility is made explicit. Similarly, Snelgrove and Liossi's aforementioned meta-synthesis of qualitative research into chronic low back pain revealed that sufferers experience overlapping implications of a psychosomatic causal process, of "imagining" one's symptoms, of "laziness", and of "seeking secondary gain" – signified together by the catchphrase "all in the mind," and united by the presumption of the sufferer's ultimate culpability (Snelgrove and Liossi, 2013, p. 292).

Causal complexity, narrative incoherence?

The *Fourth Edition* and the *Text Revision Fourth Edition* of the *DSM* – *DSM-IV* and *DSM-IV-TR* – were published in 1994 and 2000 respectively. Unlike in the equivocal *DSM III-R* classification, in *DSM-IV-TR*'s "Pain Disorder," psychological factors *must* be considered to play a significant role in the course of the disorder, although the picture that is presented is more complex than that presented in the earlier *DSM-III's* "Psychogenic Pain" classification. In *DSM-IV-TR,* psychological factors can "play a significant role" in the "onset, severity, exacerbation, or maintenance" of pain (*DSM-IV-TR*: APA, 2000, p. 485). These four words carry huge freight in terms of their implications for understanding causation and temporality of pain. To have a role in the "onset" is for "psychological factors" to have a role causally and temporally necessarily and sufficiently at the beginning of pain – as Thagard reminded us previously, these factors need not necessarily be maintained beyond the initial causal impetus. For psychological factors to play a role in pain's "severity" implies a complex and essentially non-dualistic causal process, in which these factors are understood to intensify, rather than initially cause, pain; for psychological factors to play a role in pain's "exacerbation" implies the same, although at temporally specific moments. To play a role in pain's "maintenance" implies a causal role for psychological factors with an ongoing temporal dimension, but with no causal role being required at the initiation of the disorder. By virtue of being grammatically structured as a list of alternatives, four potential scenarios are presented, each a distinct, implicit narrative. Indeed, a noun function, "psychological factors," enacts a verb function ("play a . . . role"), a grammatical structure which reproduces that of the narrative *actant* in Greimas's account, here leading to four different causal outcomes each with a distinct temporality (*DSM-IV-TR*: APA, 2000, p. 498). *DSM IV-TR* further makes clear the possibility of multiple causes by creating separate diagnostic codes: "Pain Disorder Associated with Psychological Factors," "Pain Disorder Associated with Both Psychological Factors and a General Medical Condition," and "Pain Disorder" considered to result from a "general medical condition" but where psychological factors are not considered etiological (which is "not considered a mental disorder") (*DSM-IV-TR*: APA, 2000, p. 499).

Significantly, these accounts of "Somatoform Pain Disorder" display narrative proliferation. We have seen in several sources the tendency to narrative reduction, when various causes and effects are brought together and given meaning through the allocation of a singular *actant* to bear responsibility. In *DSM IV-TR*, instead of reduction to a single *actant*, differentiated effects caused by the differentiated potential activities of *actants* are presented: as implied parallel narrative strands. Despite a presumably beneficial scope for complexity, could this proliferation, when considered in contrast to the strategies of narrative reduction that we have seen, reduce a sense of closure, and so reduce the rhetorical efficacy of this explanation? Indeed, we might wonder why narratives of psychosomatic pain in popular culture, as described throughout this volume, generally fail to reproduce such complexity and differentiation of cause. Could a differentiation and proliferation of causal responsibility contribute to an attenuation of rhetorical power, by reducing narrative and moral coherency at the level of reader response?

Controlling "psychosomatic pain": authors and *actants*

It is worth bearing this question in mind as we turn to the current *Fifth Edition* of the DSM, in which, ostensibly because of its "lack of clarity," "Somatoform Pain Disorder" fell out of favor and was removed, or at least, in a move toward narrative reduction, was combined with "Somatization Disorder" and flattened into "Somatic Symptom Disorder" (*DSM-V*: APA, 2013, p. 309). Relationships among narrative reduction, medical authority, and explanatory coherence are worth exploring here. "Somatic Symptom Disorders" are constituted by the presence of bodily symptoms, along with "abnormal thoughts, feelings, and behaviors in response to these symptoms," but with no element of psychological causation of symptoms required for diagnosis (*DSM-V*: APA, 2013, pp. 309–310). *DSM-V* notes that "a distinctive characteristic of many individuals with somatic symptoms disorder is not the somatic symptoms *per se*, but instead *the way they present and interpret them*" (*DSM-V*: APA, 2013, p. 309; emphasis added). It is clear, then, that the distress and dysfunction constitutive of the disorder are not normal responses to *pathological bodily symptoms*, but rather *pathological responses to* bodily symptoms. In this way, a basis for a diagnosable psychiatric condition is established, as the directly observable features "distress and impairment" are rendered psychopathological (*DSM-V*: APA, 2013, p. 309). This *Fifth Edition* notes that "approximately 75% of individuals previously diagnosed with hypochondriasis are subsumed under the diagnosis of somatic symptoms disorder" (*DSM-V*: APA, 2013, p. 310). It seems that in *DSM-V,* the previously established tendency found in medical and popular cultural explanations of psychosomatic pain – that of bringing into coalescence an otherwise disparate and incoherent set of issues, achieved through their reduction to a single culpable *actant* – is here extended.

The language of causation is replete with "entities" with "causal powers" or, in narrative explanations, *actants* with noun forms enacting verb functions – as previously identified as implicitly occurring in *DSM-IV-TR* through the set of "psychological factors" understood to potentially "play a significant role" in the "onset," "severity," "exacerbation," or "maintenance" of pain (*DSM-IV-TR*: APA, 2000, p. 498). By contrast, in "Somatic Symptom Disorder" the key criteria are centrally constituted by adverbial or adjectival qualifiers – "excessive," "disproportionate," "persistently" – which establish the pathological nature of the *sufferer's* interpretation of their symptoms (*DSM-V*: APA, 2013, p. 311). There are no verb functions to assign to the *sufferer/causal agent* by the terms of the definition of "Somatic Symptom Disorder," and so the adjectival qualifiers in the criteria serve to develop the *sufferer* not so much as a causal *actant* as a *character*, defined by the *manner* in which he or she does things. Significantly, the applicability of these adjectives and adverbs can only be determined through interpretations of character made by the psychiatrist. This moves further away, we would suggest, from the structure of scientific, causal explanation, and further into the territory of narrative. *DSM-V,* in focusing only on that which may be observed and putatively known by the doctor – knowledge arrived at through their interpretation and characterization of the sufferer – positions the doctor not just as *helper*, but as organizing author.

Narrative closure, according to Carroll, should ensure that "all of the questions that have been saliently posed by the narrative get answered" (2007, p. 4). In all its iterations, though in different ways, the *DSM*, rather than confronting limits to medical knowledge regarding interactions between mind and body, instead consistently elides them, and establishes criteria that allow the doctor to control closure through being able to authorize an implicit *actant* structure. Specifically, the criteria of "Psychogenic Pain Disorder," "Somatoform Pain Disorder," "Pain Disorder," and "Somatic Symptom Disorder" in each instance authorize the doctor to allocate the role of *causal agent* to the *sufferer* themselves, regardless – or perhaps because – of inconsistency and incoherency in the criteria themselves. Closure is completed as this allocation of the *causal agent* concomitantly allows the doctor to take up the role of *helper*, such that they are not only the author of, but the most powerful character within, the narrative.

Other than their potential for concatenation by a psychiatrist into a single, culpable, diagnosable *actant*, what also unifies the otherwise disparate issues or scenarios captured under the rubric "all in the mind" is that they are all, as we have written elsewhere, theoretically liable to "moral hazard" (Barker and Moseley, 2016, p. 16). This means that these scenarios – whether of pain supposedly disproportionate to known organic pathology, pain of psychogenic origin, fraudulent pain, or severe distress and dysfunction arising from pain – could all be affected by incentives built into an economic system, in a way that "organic pain," understood as a symptom of an underlying disease, for the most part cannot (Barker and Moseley, 2016, p. 16). Accordingly, such scenarios are anathema to governments and insurance companies seeking to mitigate fiscal risk by controlling "moral hazard." One strategy that may be seen to achieve such mitigation is that of insisting that pain which cannot be observed and measured, and which might be consciously or unconsciously distorted, is illegitimate (Barker and Moseley, 2016, p. 16). The previously cited qualitative research on chronic pain and stigmatization might suggest that such a sense of illegitimacy has been effectively established. The allocation to the *sufferer* of causal and (implicit or explicit) moral responsibility for their "psychosomatic pain" preserves for the allocator the power to control situations that are not fully explicable by biomedicine. Relationships between socioeconomic and political discourses, on one hand, and medical discourses on the other – and the ways in which these discourses might be mediated by power that is not only materialized, but generated, by implicit or explicit narratives – would benefit from further investigation.

Biological systems, narrative progression, and rhetorical power

As well as sharing implicit *actant* structures, popular culture narratives and medical explanations in the *DSM* can share an implicit or explicit sense of narrative progression. O'Sullivan's account of the sufferer's pathological interpretation of their symptoms corresponds to the definition of "Somatic Symptom Disorder" in *DSM-V*:

> We all perceive sensations differently, although the methods by which our bodies communicate those messages are the same for all of us. . . . Sensory and motor nerves transmit information by means of an electrical impulse. . . . The speed, integrity and size of this response can be measured and the measurements are very similar between individuals. . . . A nerve's response is standardized but how we react to the message it transmits is not. Somewhere inside our heads the message is interpreted, and it is in that interpretation that we become individuals again. Our experience of each sensation is our own. . . . We each have individual thresholds for sensation, differing pain tolerance.
>
> (O'Sullivan, 2015, p. 218)

This description, and the definition of "Somatic Symptom Disorder," both depend on a linear causal progression, as typically constitutes narrative, with its requisite structure of beginning, middle, and end. In O'Sullivan's story, the electrical discharge of a firing nerve travels to the brain, where it is uniquely interpreted by the individual. In *DSM-V*, a linear progression moving from soma to psyche is described, similar to O'Sullivan's, in the order: bodily symptom → interpretation of symptom → psychological distress → behavioral response → dysfunction in society → psychiatric diagnosis. This linear progression, in contrast to the proliferation of narrative strands in *DSM-IV-TR* with its various classificatory codes, functions as another reduction that strongly establishes closure at a narrative level.

Indeed, it is significant that the reduction and closure characteristic of many accounts of psychosomatic pain, including those in medical accounts such as "Somatic Symptom Disorder" or O'Sullivan's popularized but expert book, are at odds with complex systems-based explanations of emergent phenomena. Current pain science suggests that even the supposedly linear aspects of the transmission of nociceptive signals (that typically precipitate pain) are more in line with an emergent process, since many thousands of neural networks modulate each other and themselves in real time while under the influence of both the body's immune status and stimulus–response relationships from across all sensing domains. Even the spinal cord itself seems to be an emergent system. Current neurobiological models of pain thus suggest essential causal circularity, which seems to contradict the neat and linear story that O'Sullivan presents (see e.g. Moseley, 2013, pp. 171–173). That is, as regards pain, not only might two people interpret nociceptive signals generated by an identical noxious stimulus quite differently, as O'Sullivan notes, but, if we follow contemporary neurobiological models, it seems that such individual interpretations always have the potential to affect the body's physiological processing of nociceptive signals at the spinal cord itself, which can lead to differences in the levels of nociceptive signaling ultimately reaching the brain (for a description of such "descending modulation" see e.g. Butler and Moseley, 2014, p. 73; Cambier, 1993, p. 356). Further, not only does brain activity affect sensory processing in the spinal cord, but recent work on the idea of a "cortical body matrix" suggests that the very mechanisms by which we feel things seem to have specific effects on the body itself, helping to maintain homeostasis (see e.g. Moseley *et al.*, 2012). Indeed, it seems that subjective symptoms can physiologically affect "objective" signs.

The causal circularity between brain and spinal cord, between mind and body, evident in these neurobiological accounts suggests that pain should not be understood in dualistic or linear terms, and that causal responsibility for pain and its severity is complex and dispersed. Such dispersal would seem to oppose narrative reduction. Identifying a singular, indivisible *actant* – to whom responsibility for a set of non-equivalent and at times inconsistent effects may be imputed – achieves coherence through a unity of causal and moral closure, and answers the implicit question, *Who or what is responsible?* As this chapter has argued, such a structuring principle, and the allocation of culpability that it permits, is generative of rhetorical power, with the potential to serve political or economic narratives as well as medical authority. To conclude with a series of questions: might complex systems-based explanations of pain, that disperse causal responsibility, simultaneously disperse implicit moral responsibility, such that the question – *Who or what is responsible?* – cannot be met with a reassuring or easily manipulable answer? Given that the medical explanations previously considered authorize the maintenance of control by the doctor over "psychosomatic pain," and given the near impossibility of obtaining knowledge of exact causal interactions in a complex system, could explanations assuming a dispersal of causal responsibility also disperse such power and control, potentially destigmatizing the sufferer and breaking down distinctions between "psychosomatic" and "organic" pain? The use of *actant* structures has been shown to enhance rhetorical power but can be readily deployed to serve vested interests; on the other hand, must the potential benefits of biologically precise, systems-based explanations be accompanied by a loss of narrative coherence and rhetorical power? If so, the practical and ethical balancing of these tensions remains a crucial and unfulfilled task.

References

Abbott, H.P. (2008). *The Cambridge Introduction to Narrative* (2nd edn). Cambridge: Cambridge University Press.

American Psychiatric Association. (1980). *Diagnostic and Statistical Manual of Mental Disorders, 3rd Edition*. Washington, DC: Author.

American Psychiatric Association. (1987). *Diagnostic and Statistical Manual of Mental Disorders, 3rd Edition, Revised*. Washington, DC: Author.

American Psychiatric Association. (1994). *Diagnostic and Statistical Manual of Mental Disorders, 4th Edition*. Washington, DC: Author.

American Psychiatric Association. (2000). *Diagnostic and Statistical Manual of Mental Disorders, 4th Edition, Text Revision*. Washington, DC: Author.

American Psychiatric Association. (2013). *Diagnostic and Statistical Manual of Mental Disorders, 5th Edition*. Washington, DC: Author.

Aronowitz, R.A. (2004). When do symptoms become a disease? In A.L. Caplan, J.J. McCartney, and D.A. Sisti (eds), *Health, Disease, and Illness: Concepts in Medicine* (pp. 65–75). Washington, DC: Georgetown University Press.

Barker, S. and Moseley, G.L. (2016). The difficult problem: Chronic pain and the politics of care. *Australian Quarterly, 87*(3), 8–17. Available atwww.aips.net.au/aq-magazine/current-edition/. ISSN: 1443–3605.

Boorse, C. (2004). On the distinction between disease and illness. In A.L. Caplan, J.J. McCartney, and D.A. Sisti (eds), *Health, Disease, and Illness: Concepts in Medicine* (pp. 77–89). Washington, DC: Georgetown University Press.

Brémond, C. (1973). *Logique du récit*. Paris: Éditions du Seuil.

Bury, M. (1982). Chronic illness as biographical disruption. *Sociology of Health and Illness*, *4*(2), 167–182. Available at http://doi.org/10.1111/1467-9566.ep11339939.

Butler, D. and Moseley, G.L. (2014). *Explain Pain* (2nd edn). Adelaide: Noigroup Publications.

Cambier, J. (1993). A modern view. In R. Rey, *History of Pain*, translated by L.E. Wallace, J.A. Cadden, and W. Cadden. Paris: La Découverte.

Carroll, N. (2007). Narrative closure. *Philosophical Studies, 135*, 1–15. doi 10.1007/s11098-007-9097-9.

Diagnosis. (2016). In *Oxford English Dictionary*. Available at www.oed.com/view/Entry/51836?redirectedFrom=diagnosis#eid (accessed July 20, 2016).

Dowling, W. C. (2011). *Ricoeur on Time and Narrative: An Introduction to Temps et récit*. Notre Dame, IN.: University of Notre Dame Press.

Good, M-J. D., Brodwin, P. E., Good, B. J., and Kleinman, A. (1994). *Pain as Human Experience: An Anthropological Perspective*. Berkeley: University of California Press.

Greimas, A. J. (1983). *Structural Semantics: An Attempt at a Method*, translated by D. McDowell, R. Schleifer, and A. Velie. Lincoln: University of Nebraska Press.

Hucklenbroich, P. (2014). "Disease entity" as the key theoretical concept of medicine. *The Journal of Medicine and Philosophy*, *39*(6), 609–633. Available at http://doi.org/10.1093/jmp/jhu040.

Karhausen, L. R. (2000). Causation: The elusive grail of epidemiology. *Medicine, Health Care and Philosophy*, *3*(1), 59–67. Available at http://doi.org/10.1023/A:1009970730507.

Mel' uk, I. (2015). *Semantics: From Meaning to Text*, edited by D. Beck and A. Polguère. Philadelphia, PA: John Benjamins Publishing Company.

Moseley, G. L. (2013). Reconceptualising pain according to modern pain science. *Physical Therapy Reviews, 12*(3), 169–178. doi: 10.1179/108331907X223010.

Moseley, G. L., Gallace, A., and Spence, C. (2012). Body illusions in health and disease: Physiological and clinical perspectives and the concept of a cortical "body matrix." *Neuroscience and Biobehavioral Reviews, 36*(2012), 34–46. doi:10.1016/j.neubiorev.2011.03.3013.

O'Sullivan, S. (2015). *It's All in Your Head: True Stories of Imaginary Illness*. New York: Random House.

O'Toole, M. T. (ed.). (2013). *Mosby's Medical Dictionary*. St. Louis, MO: Elsevier.

Pelletier, K. R. (1977). *Mind as Healer, Mind as Slayer: A Holistic Approach to Preventing Stress Disorders*. New York: Dell.

Propp, V. (1968). *Morphology of the Folktale*, translated by D. Scott. Austin: Texas University Press.

Snelgrove, S. and Liossi, C. (2013). Living with chronic low back pain: A metasynthesis of qualitative research. *Chronic Illness*, *9*(4), 283–301. Available at http://doi.org/10.1177/1742395313476901.

Sontag, S. (1991). *Illness as Metaphor and AIDS and its Metaphors*. London: Penguin.

Thagard, P. (1998). Explaining disease: Correlations, causes, and mechanisms. *Minds and Machines*, *8*(1), 61–78. Available at http://doi.org/10.1023/A:1008286314688.

7 Medicalstudentitis as a rite of passage in popular literature

Maria Tutorskaya

Prologue

One day, I saw one of my first-year medical students in tears after class. When I asked if she was okay, she said no, handing me her blood test result – there were increased white blood cells, mainly monocytes and lymphocytes. She added that she had already examined herself, found that her lymph nodes were enlarged, read about such symptoms in the textbook, and decided without a doubt that it must be leukemia. I tried my best to cheer her up and to convince her to just see her doctor. When I saw her next, she said that it was not cancer, merely infectious mononucleosis, and that she felt stupid about her fears.

Introduction

In this chapter, I would like to emphasize several aspects of the condition Medicalstudentitis as an example of a psychosomatic disorder, a condition that involves both mind (psyche) and body (soma). Medicalstudentitis, also known as medical students' disease or syndrome, is defined as "A constellation of signs and symptoms which a medical student believes he or she has while learning about a particular disease in medical school; a collection of psychosomatic symptoms resulting from the study of a disorder as a medical student."[1] The purpose of this chapter is to investigate narratives about this disease and to analyze the condition as an example of a rite of passage. I will examine excerpts from novels written by Russian and American writers, in particular *The Memoirs of a Physician* by Russian physician Vikenty Veresaev first published in 1901, and *Doctors* by American writer Erich Segal published about 90 years later in 1988. In these novels Medicalstudentitis is depicted very similarly as an initiation to the medical profession.

I will use an anthropological perspective and methodology, starting with the concept of the rite of passage as defined by the French anthropologist Arnold van Gennep and his follower, British cultural anthropologist Victor Turner. Van Gennep's major work, *The Rite of Passage* (1909), was devoted to the "initiation [as a] ceremony or period of instruction with which a new member is admitted to an organization or to knowledge" (p. 10). He considered that it is legitimate to single out rites of passage as "ceremonies that celebrate an individual's transition from one status to another within a given society" (p. 10). These rites could be subdivided into three steps: rites of separation (preliminary rites), transition rites (liminal rites), and rites of incorporation and reassimilation (postliminal rites). Van Gennep emphasized that there is such "incompatibility between the profane and the sacred worlds that man cannot pass from one to the other without going through an intermediate stage" and that the "life of the individual in any society is a series of passages from one age to another and from one occupation to another" (pp. 1, 3). Sixty years later, Victor Turner, in his book, *The Ritual Process* (1969), expanded the understanding of this stage of initiation, applying the concept of liminality not only to individuals but also to the experience of groups and whole societies. He pointed out that liminalities are "necessarily ambiguous" and that one's "sense of identity dissolves" during the liminal passage, revealing uncertainty and "possibility of new perspectives" at the same time (p. 195).

I argue that going through medical students' disease in the fictional narratives mentioned above may be seen as "traversing several boundaries" and an initiation to the profession that could be split into the stages articulated by Arnold van Gennep. The preliminary phase is related to the separation of medical students from the lay world in the medical school. At the second, liminal, stage, the future doctor experiences hypochondria, soul-searching, and a confrontation of mortality. In the third, postliminal, stage the transformation from the lay world to the professional medical community occurs.

I am examining this condition through the lens of literature because, by developing a critical discourse about literature and medicine, we may achieve a more holistic view of the disease: its causes, how students go through it, and ultimately how it affects doctors. Paul Atkinson suggests that "Becoming a 'hypochondriac' may be an occupational hazard for those who are in process of becoming medical experts" (quoted in Baur, 1989, p. 170). Harold Nicolson asserts that "All creative writers are hypochondriacs, since those of them who do not worry about the state of their bodies are certain to worry about the state of their minds" (Nicolson, 1947, p. 709). Both stated that medical students' disease –hypochondriasis – is an occupational hazard shared in doctoring and writing alike (quoted in Baur, 1989, p. 1). In citing these epigraphs together, Baur accentuates the connection between literature and medicine; similarly, it makes sense to look at these issues together here in this chapter.

There have been no specialized studies of medical students' disease in popular literature, nor has the condition been analyzed as a rite of passage either. However, we can observe many instances where physicians and writers have tried to analyze this condition in narrative – whether novels,[2] autobiographies, or short stories. I will try to show the writer's understanding of the meanings of the possible causes of medical students' disease, how medical students go through this experience, and how it influences both their personality and future professional career.

Understanding medical students' disease through the lens of medical research

Medicalstudentitis is also known as medical students' disease, hypochondriasis of medical students, third-year syndrome, second-year syndrome, or intern syndrome. Students with this condition perceive themselves to be experiencing the symptoms of the disease(s) they are studying. Medical student syndrome has been assessed in several, admittedly qualitative, medical research studies. According to Hunter andcolleagues (1964), approximately 70 percent of medical students had "groundless medical fears during their studies" (p. 147). Woods and colleagues (1966) indicated that 78.8 percent of 33 randomly chosen medical first-year students demonstrated a "history of medical student disease" (p. 785). The first controlled research, conducted by Kellner and colleagues (1986), matched 60 medical students with 60 law students. The study revealed that hypochondriacal fears did not differ significantly between the two groups, and that law students worry about their health just as much as their medical student peers (p. 487). Moss-Morris and Petrie (2001) then matched first-, second-, and third-year medical students with law students and supported the separation of medical students' disease into perceptual and emotional components. Their findings showed that first-year medical students have the highest level of health anxiety, compared to law students and medical students in the second and the third year of learning. The researchers stated: "Medical students' disease can also be used as a personally relevant example in teaching how patients make sense of symptoms" (p. 724), urging future doctors toward self-reflection and introspection. The authors suggested that students' awareness about the nature of their health scares could offset their irrationality and become useful teaching cases in the medical classroom. Most recently, Azuri andcolleagues (2010, p. 273) concluded that:

> "Medical students' disease" should be regarded as a psychosomatic syndrome depending on the years of learning. By breaking it down into its components, one can better characterize it and predict its onset. By defining it as a normal process, one can assist in guiding medical students to reduce their level of anxiety and distress.

These researchers encourage medical educators to consider this condition as "a double-edged sword" with the potential to simultaneously distress students and help them to cope with the studying process.

Medical study of students' health anxiety started only in the 1960s, so it could be considered as a rather "poorly characterized" and poorly studied illness that has no effective and proven treatment (Salkovskis and Howes, 1998, p. 1332). However, as with many issues of medicine, it has also been treated in figurative and poetic disguise in great works of literature. Writers have long created the image of the disease in light of their own medical schooling, observation of students' feelings and impressions, teaching, and the patient's experience. In these literary sources the causes of the medical students' disease were related to the huge amount of information about the variety of illnesses for which they are responsible, obsessively scrutinized rote learning from textbooks, and lack of diagnostic experience. The most common example of hypochondria provoked by medical knowledge in popular literature and an image of the disease as it exists in the public mind in contemporary Russia was given at the end of the nineteenth century by a British writer, Jerome K. Jerome, in *Three Men in a Boat* (1889). Jerome's hero plodded conscientiously through the 26 letters of a medical encyclopedia, and the only malady he could conclude he had *not* got was housemaid's knee, reaffirming that "Knowledge without practice makes but half an artist" (p. 3).

Preliminality: separation rites

I will interpret the precursor stage of Medicalstudentitis as a separation (preliminal) rite which displaces students from their previous station. At the start of the twentieth century (1901), Vikentiy Veresaev published his semi-autobiographical novel *The Memoirs of a Physician*. The book made him famous immediately. Veresaev dealt with such issues as medical education, the doctor–patient relationship, human experimentation, and medical errors. The book became the subject of intense discussions in the professional and popular spheres both nationally and internationally.

Veresaev enrolled in the medical faculty at Dorpat University (University of Tartu) in 1888. In his *Memoirs* he describes feeling lonely and disconnected, not belonging to the world that surrounds him. As a newcomer he recognizes the striking comparison between vigorous Saint Petersburg – the city where he got his Master's degree – and quiet Dorpat, the town that lives only for the university. Moreover, he discovers that students are divided into local associations – seven corporations in which most students are included. Those that are barred from membership, like Veresaev, are called "wild" (Veresaev, 1961, p. 72), and thus set apart both from their family ambiance and the student community. In addition to this separation, things that seemed common to him before, such as his own body and eating, are reviewed and reconsidered. Veresaev finds that the phenomena which surround and fill him, and which he

> contemplated before with the eyes of a savage, now became plain and comprehensible. . . . Every day, every lecture brought new "discoveries" in their wake and I am astounded to learn, for instance, that the meat I ate in the form of beef-steaks and cutlets was mysterious matter called "muscle," which hitherto my imagination had vaguely pictured as balls of greyish thread.
>
> (Veresaev, 1961, p. 2)

Several decades later, Erich Segal, a professor of Greek and Latin literature at Harvard University, made a comprehensive study concerning medical education and practice in his novel *Doctors* (1988). While Veresaev discusses both his loneliness and the "discoveries" he made which formed a new outlook on life and self-awareness, Segal's portrayal of the Harvard Medical School class of 1962 represents the isolation of medical students as a traumatic experience.

Both writers have recourse to allegorical and allusive epithets that reference magic and ritual more than the prosaic course of life. Segal's choice of opening epigraph, a quote from physician-poet William Carlos Williams' poem "Spring and All," sets readers on the path to the preliminal rite and their rebirth as "novices" (Williams, 2011, p. 183). Williams, the doctor, poet, and short story writer, establishes a relationship between the uncertainty and changes that together accompany "entering the new world." The strophe "By the road to the contagious hospital" may be interpreted as a metaphorical path to medicine. Medical students are "leafless vines," which seem "lifeless in appearance" but which have a strong potential to be soon defined: "sluggish dazed spring approaches." Segal invokes Williams's poem (not to mention the example offered by his career) to set a precedent for Barney Livingston and Laura Castellano – the heroes of the novel – who also use metaphor when they share their dread of becoming doctors. They joke about needing an incantation, an "open sesame to Med School" and entering a new cryptic world. Through the novel's plot twist they break connections with the rest of the world, even their parents, as they enter medical school (p. 230). In Turner's terminology, these first-year students are detached from their "earlier fixed point in the social structure" or "a set of cultural conditions" and fall into a gap between the profane and sacred worlds when entering university.

Liminality: transition rites

When Veresaev was in his third year of study (1891), he conceived of an idea of a medical student's diary to record his expectations about working in the clinic, and, finding "a lot of interesting and characteristic going on there," to write about these impressions. Some of the notes from this diary were used as a foundation for *The Memoirs of a Physician,* completed in 1901. Veresaev describes how the stress which medical students face, their first "date" with patients, and their first diagnostic experiences all combine to provoke hypochondria. Going from formulas and abstract concepts to real-life situations tempts the hero of the novel to look for symptoms in himself:

A small mole under my left arm-pit, without any apparent cause, suddenly began to increase in size and become painful. I was afraid to believe the evidence of my senses, but it grew and grew, and hurt me more every day. At last the swelling attained the size of a hazel-nut. There was no room for further doubt: the mole had developed into a sarcoma, that terrible melanosarcoma which generally originates from innocent-looking beauty spots. I went to attend the consulting hours of our professor of surgery, feeling as if I were about to have a final interview with the hangman.

"Professor, I believe . . . I have a sarcoma of the arm," I said in an unsteady voice.

The professor scrutinized me attentively. "Are you a medical student of the third course?"

"Yes."

"Show me your sarcoma!"

I undressed. The professor removed the growth by severing its narrow stem with a pair of scissors.

"Your sleeve had merely irritated the mole, nothing more. Take your sarcoma with you as a keep-sake!" he said, smiling good-naturedly and handing me a small fleshy pellet. I went away happy, although much ashamed, and I felt abashed at my childish apprehensiveness.

(Veresaev, 1901, p. 13)

The type of medical students' disease that Veresaev shows in this quote appears later in Erich Segal's *Doctors*. Diligent engagement combined with the absence of real-world practice nudge students to "try on" the symptoms of studied diseases. Erich Segal shows medical students' disease not just as the personal experience of a single anxious student, but as a kind of epidemic of mass hysteria:

It's very common among medical students. Nosophobia literally means "fear of diseases". It's caused by having to memorize the Merck Manual, which has every kind of bizarre illness that ever existed. We'll all of us have a touch of noso during the year. . . . I mean there is an epidemic in our whole class and the most amazing part is that no two people have the same complaint. For example, Laura believes she is suffering from endometriosis, that shows that she's got more sense than Lance because it's benign and can be cured by surgery. In fact, this noso craze has made everybody in the goddam class a hypochondriac.

(Segal, 1988, p. 244)

Segal indicates that hypochondria touches upon almost the whole cohort. Some students routinely develop vivid delusions of having the "disease of the week" (Baars, 1997, p. 104). For others, every symptom and malaise becomes a sign of cancer:

- I've got testicular teratoma.
- Have you seen a doctor?
- I don't have to. I've got every symptom in the goddam textbook. And what clinches it is that the condition peaks in twenty-four-year-old guys. My birthday was only last week and I felt the first twinge when I was cutting the cake. And I've checked it.

(Segal, 1988, p. 243)

Similarly, after having the "cancer experience," Veresaev's doesn't feel himself to be on safe ground. Veresaev shows that he is not reassured by the case and soon afterwards becomes nosophobic of diabetes. He compares his symptoms of physical manifestations of anxiety with the symptoms in the textbook and even devises tests for himself. He has the courage to seek reassurance and consults with his professor of therapeutics. And he gets the same professional advice from his mentor as with his cancer scare:

Soon afterwards I began to notice that something abnormal was taking place within me: I experienced a general lassitude and distaste for work, I lost my appetite and I constantly suffered from thirst. I lost flesh too, and every now and then abscesses formed on different parts of my body; I passed water very abundantly; I tested it for sugar – it contained none. All these symptoms pointed to diabetes insipidus. In deep dejection I perused the chapter devoted to that disease in Strumpell's text-book. I went to our professor of therapeutics. Without telling him of my fears, I simply detailed my symptoms. As I proceeded the professor's brows contracted more and more.

He cut me short. "You suppose that you have diabetes insipidus. It is very praise-worthy that you should have studied Strumpell so painstakingly; you have not omitted a single symptom. I hope you will be as well up in the subject when the examinations come round. Smoke less, eat more, take more exercise, and leave off thinking of diabetes."

(Veresaev, 1901, p. 14)

Without a shadow of a doubt the professor recognizes the disease and writes a prescription. He is concerned that the cause of the disease lies in "painstaking studies" but he also mentions contributing factors such as smoking, junk food, and lack of exercise. The type of chronic worrying that the hero has could be considered as an argument for the idea that coping with stress and pressure exerted by forthcoming examinations (stress exacerbated by unhealthy living), combined with witnessing the suffering of patients in clinics, brings the future caregiver into the uncertain, fearful world of pain and disability. Arthur Kleinman, psychiatrist and anthropologist, defined hypochondria as "a chronic condition in which the patient persists in his nosophobia in spite of medical evidence to the contrary" (Kleinman, 1988, p. 194). Veresaev placed extra emphasis on the irony: medical students have no lack of medical evidence but are helplessly subjective because of inexperience and their own ambiguous status. As Montgomery (2006, p. 5) observes, "Medicine's success relies on the physician's capacity for clinical judgment" and that "medicine remains an interpretive practice." Through the example of their protagonists, Vikentiy Veresaev and Erich Segal point out that interpretive practice finds an unlikely beginning from the habit of false self-diagnosis.

The preceding examples from Veresaev and Segal reveal that the conditions most suspected and dreaded by medical students are predominantly the deadliest diseases, above all cancer. Fear of death and the ensuing confrontation of mortality is inherent to those on the threshold who are "neither here nor there" (Turner, 1969, p. 232). Van Gennep offered interpretations of the significance of such rites of passage "as forms of social regeneration, based on such natural symbols as death and rebirth"; and Turner further pointed out that "liminality is frequently likened to death" (Turner, 1969, p. 95). Characteristically, in the case of medical students, that reflection on *memento mori* is especially intensified, as they live through one imaginary fatal disease after another in combination with the dissection of human cadavers in Gross Anatomy. Segal's students mark the paradox that before "preserving the living they must first preserve the dead" (Segal, 1988, p. 93).

An ability to "take this part" is widely accepted as an initiation into medicine (Belling, 2012, p. 112); however, I would argue that dissection is a rather more distinctive component of liminality than the passage on the whole. An integral feature of the liminal, intermediate stage is the introduction to new actions and knowledge, a part of the typical sequence of stages that leads to obtaining a new social status. Dissection is one of the good examples of action that becomes sacred to the initiate, forbidden to the profane layperson (Durkheim, 2001, p. 52). An acquaintance with a variety of viruses, bacteria, and somatic diseases is another. These components of the rite shake students' understanding of the world. Fears of physical illness and bodily vulnerability appear in conjunction with the study of pathology and pathophysiology, and result in an understanding of the fragility of one's own health and the limited possibilities of medicine. Then, the first clinical experience and the interaction with suffering patients causes the students to reflect on the boundary between their own life and death, health and disease, causing physiological distress through that involvement. The experience of medical students' disease may be individualized and depends on the type of personality, temperament, or situation of the student – but the cause of the disease is the same.

Postliminality: incorporation rites

Passing through the stages of acceptance of the disease (denial or shock, anger, bargaining, depression, acceptance) may be considered as a ritual or social formation in a doctor's world and may be compared to shamanic sickness. Similar to the way in which shamans establish connection with the spiritual world, allopathic students, through medicalstudentitis, become doctors. Understanding the falsity of their own diagnosis and analysis of their error comes after acceptance, not to mention a better understanding of the profession and medicine in its entirety.

Medical pedagogy seems incomplete without experiencing the self-suggestion and hypnotic effects of clinical practice. Medicalstudentitis is perceived by some physicians as one of the stages of learning, like overcoming the fear of dissecting, getting used to the smell of formalin, and remembering complex Latin terms. The condition is romanticized by doctors in literature as one of the fondest memories of their times as a student. Baur and Atkinson state that becoming a hypochondriac may be an "occupational hazard for those who are in process of becoming medical experts" (quoted in Baur, 1989, p. 170). In their perception it is "not a somatizing response to the stress of medical school but a valid cognitive reaction to the new knowledge, and to new ways of reading." Salkovskis and Howes (1998) conceptualized it as a mild form of health anxiety or transient occupational hypochondriasis. It is seen as the liminal stage that is not just a reaction to early medical education but an inherent part of that education, an active step in the formation of physicians. The medical community not only considers medicalstudentitis to be "a normal perceptual process, rather than a form of hypochondriasis" but even suggests using this condition as a "personally relevant example in teaching about how patients make sense of symptoms" (Moss-Morris and Petrie, 2001, p. 724). From this point, anxiety turns into a kind of self-modeling tool that is included in the educational process and by extension the medical habitus.

It is important to note that liminality, as a "condition of doubt" (Belling 2012, p. 17), is not only bounded with health; in addition, this general anxiety leads initiates to experience a skeptical, but necessary, doubt in both their own potential and capacity, as well as in all their once habitual, foundational assumptions about the world. Students tend to "believe, without any reason, that they know absolutely everything, or, also without any grounds, they start to think that they do not know anything" (German, 1964, p. 425). The definition of self and professional allegiance is severely challenged. Therefore, students' postliminal rite of passage includes acceptance of their future profession, including a profound awareness that "all flesh is grass,"[3] and that errors and malpractice (their own in particular) are always possible. Reappraisal and reinterpretation of medicine is a part of incorporation. Considering the indeterminacy of science in treating certain diseases, students may become more and more impregnated with a species of absolute medical nihilism, confessing that "all our doctoring was merely humbug"; but they can just as easily change their uncompromising stance in a moment after facing successful healing in the treatment of critically ill patients:

> You are a physician, therefore you ought to be able to recognize and cure every ill; if, however, you are powerless to do so, and it follows that you must be a quack. . . . From that day forward, my attitude towards medicine underwent a radical change. On commencing its study I expected it to accomplish everything; seeing that medicine could not do all, I concluded that it could do nothing. Now, however, I saw how much it could still do, and that "much" filled me with reliance in, and respect for, that science I had so recently despised from the bottom of my soul.
>
> (Veresaev, 1901, p. 47)

Notably, Veresaev's hero overcome his nihilism and was very optimistic about "how much medicine he could still do" (Veresaev, 1901, p. 47). His comprehension is influenced by a strong belief in finding a cure for every illness through the scientific progress that developed following the discovery of the germ theory of disease in the late nineteenth century. By contrast, Segal's students doubt medicine as well but are more skeptical in their conclusions after "reconvalescence":

> When the mass hysteria had finally abated, the students drew a lesson from this experience. But unfortunately it was one that would actually harm them in later life. For they, whose primary training would be in observation and detection of signs and symptoms in others, had blunted their own powers to perceive true illness in themselves. Besides, a real physician almost never seeks another doctor's help. For they all are painfully aware of just how little anybody understands about curing the sick.
>
> (Segal, 1988, p. 245)

In acquiring professional identity they are becoming aware of the limits of their own capabilities and opportunities, and of medicine itself. Their skepticism reflects the trends of the time – the sunset of the "Golden Age of Medicine" and strenuous opposition against doctors in society (Brandt and Gardner, 2000, p. 22). Although published in the late 1980s, Segal reflects on an earlier period, following the class of 1962 at Harvard Medical School; his heroes are led to question medicine, reflecting the larger historical trend of a distrust of medicine's potency as an objective science and its authority, and the rejection of the paternalistic model of the physician–patient relationship. This major cognitive shift in students' aggregation toward the profession in turn results in the formation of a new relationship between themselves and others which is significant because it shapes their meaning-making, and nudges them toward critical thinking.

Conclusion

For a long time, medicalstudentitis was unknown and not of interest to non-specialists. In modern medicine, in part due to informed patient consent and an effort to make the clinical encounter more inclusive and less hierarchical, reading of medical narratives by patients has become more common. A century ago, hypochondria was considered grotesque, but today, every other person could say that they have had experiences similar to those of medical students. The medicalization of society has led to a proliferation of self-examination, self-diagnosis, and even self- or home treatment. Millions can easily search the Internet for information about any disease and come away believing that they may have those symptoms.

In *The Memoirs of a Physician* by Vikenty Veresaev and in *Doctors* by Erich Segal, medical students' disease is represented as a turning point, a rite of passage, which marks the entrance into a professional medical world. In contradistinction to the traditional rites of passage, like transition from childhood or adolescence to adulthood, Veresaev's and Segal's students undergoing medicalstudentitis don't change their official status. Nonetheless, the process changes their perception, their worldview, and their identity, and increases their feelings of affiliation toward the "mysteries" of medicine. Furthermore, these literary artists present this condition evoking empathy and understanding that could not be aroused by medical research papers and textbooks dealing with symptoms and treatment methods. Accordingly, these works deserve a place in the list of recommended literature for the kinds of literature and medicine courses increasingly studied by premed and medical students. Their practical value (I define medicine as a practice, following Montgomery's arguments[4]) could not only meet curricular goals for both the medical humanities and medical education, but could also become a kind of prevention and therapy for stressed and disoriented students.

Rita Charon – founder of the program in narrative medicine at Columbia University – accentuates the significance of self-reflection and stories in medical education. She states that analyzing narratives and reflective writing stimulates "professionals' willingness and skill to examine students' own experiences and to make sense of their own journeys, not for solipsistic reasons but for the sake of improving the care they can deliver," thereby equipping proto-doctors with "compassion's prerequisites" (Charon, 2006, pp. 66, 27). According to this intention, the humanizing benefits of literature might not only contribute to students' cultural *niveau* but could lead to a more empathetic and compassionate practice of medicine.

It is worth noting that medical students' disease is one of the first challenges that doctors face during their career. The perceptual and emotional components of personal insight depend on many conditions: personality, age, gender, race, and personal circumstances. Even time is a factor: the onset of medical students' disease depends on the syllabus and one's year in medical school. Both researchers and writers hold the view that self-diagnosis, even when it results in misdiagnosis, as it frequently does, helps future doctors in their professional development and is an active step in the formation of physicians.

In conclusion, I would like to mention (following Van Gennep) that "The transition from one state to another is a serious step which could not be accomplished without special precautions." Thus, advance warning of this trial could help students reduce stress and anxiety. The experience of hypochondria could provide valuable knowledge and help in understanding how patients make sense of their symptoms, and it could teach empathy and develop critical analysis abilities. Finally, the student's self-suggestion may lead to the early diagnosis of health problems that actually exist either in herself or in her patients.

Notes

1 Medical students' disease. In *Segen's Medical Dictionary*. Huntingdon Valley: Farlex Inc., 2012. Available at Medical-dictionary.thefreedictionary.com (accessed December 10, 2015).
2 Notably, such hypochondriacs were described in Conan Doyle's short stories, *Cancer Ward* by Aleksandr Solzhenitsyn, and Veniamin Kaverin's and Vasily Aksyonov's novels.
3 Old Testament, Isaiah 40:6.
4 Montgomery (2006) defines medicine not as an exact or hard science, but as an interpretive practice that is guided by clinical judgment. She also states that stress among med school newcomers is related to the uncertainty, variability, and ambiguity they encounter in medical knowledge instead of "facts" and universal algorithms for treatment that they expected to obtain.

References

Azuri, J., Ackshota, N., and Vinker, S. (2010). Reassuring the medical students' disease – Health related anxiety among medical students. *Medical Teacher*, *32*(7), e270–e275. Available at http://dx.doi.org/10.3109/0142159x.2010.490282.

Baars, B. (1997). *In the Theater of Consciousness*. New York: Oxford University Press.

Baur, S. (1989). *Hypochondria*. Berkeley: University of California Press.

Belling, C. (2012). *A Condition of Doubt*. New York: Oxford University Press.

Brandt, A.M. and Gardner, M. (2000). The golden age of medicine? In R. Cooter and J. Pickstone, *Medicine in the Twentieth Century* (pp. 21–37). Amsterdam: Harwood Academic.

Charon, R. (2006). *Narrative Medicine*. Oxford: Oxford University Press.

Durkheim, E. (2001). *The elementary forms of religious life.* Oxford: Oxford University Press.

Gennep, A. van (1960 [1909]). *The rites of passage.* Chicago: University of Chicago Press.

German, I. *The Cause You Serve.* Moscow: Foreign Languages Pub. House, 1964.

Hunter, R., Lohrenz, J., and Schwartzman, A. (1964). Nosophobia and hypochondriasis in medical students. *The Journal of Nervous and Mental Disease*, *139*(2), 147–152. Available at http://dx.doi.org/10.1097/00005053-196408000-00008.

Jerome, K. J. (2012). *Three Men in a Boat.* Dayboro: Emereo Publishers.

Kellner, R. (1986). Hypochondriacal fears and beliefs in medical and law students. *Archives of General Psychiatry*, *43*(5), 487. Available at http://dx.doi.org/10.1001/archpsyc.1986.01800050093012.

Kleinman, A. (1988). *The Illness Narratives.* New York: Basic Books.

Montgomery, K. (2006). *How Doctors Think.* Oxford: Oxford University Press.

Moss-Morris, R. and Petrie, K. (2001). Redefining medical students' disease to reduce morbidity. *Medical Education*, *35*(8), 724–728. Available at http://dx.doi.org/10.1046/j.1365-2923.2001.00958.xhttp://dx.doi.org/10.1046/j.1365-2923.2001.00958.x.

Nicolson, H. (1947). The health of authors. *The Lancet*, *250*(6481), 709–714.

Pratt, C. (2012, March 3). Shaman's sickness, initiation and the calling. Available athttp://whyshamanismnow.com/2012/03/shaman's-sickness-initiation-and-the-calling/.

Salkovskis, P. and Howes, O. (1998). Health anxiety in medical students. *The Lancet*, *351*(9112), 1332. Available at http://dx.doi.org/10.1016/s0140-6736(05)79059-0.

Segal, E. (1988). *Doctors.* New York: Bantam (Penguin/Random House).

Turner, V. W. (1969). *The Ritual Process: Structure and Anti-structure.* Chicago, IL: Aldine Publishers.

Veresaev, V. V. (1916). *The Memoirs of a Physician*, ed. H. Pleasants. New York: A.A. Knopf. (Original work published 1901.)

Veresaev, V. V. (1961). *Sobraniesochinenij v pjati tomah.* Moscow: Pravda.

Williams, W. C. (2011). "Spring and All". New York: New Directions Publishing.

Woods, S., Natterson, J., and Silverman, J. (1966). Medical students' disease. *Academic Medicine*, *41*(8), 785–790. Available at http://dx.doi.org/10.1097/00001888-196608000-00006.

8 Women with long-term exhaustion in fictional literature

A comparative approach

Olaug S. Lian, Catherine Robson,
and Hilde Bondevik

Introduction

The main theme of this chapter is depictions of long-term exhaustion, a severe form of tiredness, in historical and contemporary fictional literature. Tiredness and exhaustion are real both in a biological and an experiential sense: the phenomena entail experiences of biological processes that go on in the human body. In this chapter, however, it is the cultural dimension of these phenomena that interests us. Although our perceptions are individually and subjectively perceived, they are prefigured by the sociocultural contexts in which we are situated, and therefore infused with culturally defined norms and values. These norms and values are generated through interactions among human beings, and therefore vary between time and place. Culturally and historically contingent norms on exhaustion define rules about who has permission to be exhausted, and when, where, and how we are allowed to express it (Widerberg, 2005). These perceptions are gendered: men and women seem to handle tiredness differently and the (stereotyped) masculine response – to pull yourself together and "handle it like a man" (Widerberg, 2005, p.111) – is perceived as the culturally more legitimate form in our culture, where tiredness is seen as a sign of weakness, and the normative ideals are energy, toughness, strength, and endurance (ibid.).

Cultural norms and values on how to think about and deal with experiences of exhaustion are expressed, created, maintained, and challenged in a complex interplay among different actors operating in social fields, not only in day-to-day interactions between human beings, but also in powerful fields such as the medical system and the field of fiction and the popular press.[1] One way to explore cultural norms surrounding expressions of exhaustion, then, is to study literary texts. Through creative and artistic expressions, literary texts depict, convey, and create culturally and historically contingent interpretations of social realities. Sometimes these expressions also represent wide-ranging cultural critiques of these interpreted realities (Schaffner, 2016). Literary texts are mediators between the individual subject and the larger group (Thompson, 2015), and studying these texts in a sociocultural context may help us unveil the intricate interplay between social structures and individual actors (Antoft *et al.*, 2010). Building on this assumption, commonly found in the sociology of literature, combined with a historical

sociological approach (Abrams, 1982), we explore culturally and historically contingent norms and values related to long-term exhaustion.

We approach this task through an analysis of three literary texts, all written by
prominent authors and regarded as key literary works of their time: Gustav Flaubert's *Emma Bovary* (1857), Charlotte Perkins Gilman's *The Yellow Wallpaper*
(1892), and Sue Townsend's *The Woman Who Went to Bed for a Year* (2012). Our
main questions are these: how is severe long-term exhaustion portrayed in modern
contemporary literary texts compared to nineteenth-century texts? In what ways
are these texts related to medical constructions of illness, disease, and diagnosis
involving these experiences, and the *Zeitgeist* of their time? And how can literary representations of this ailment serve to enlighten contemporary debates about
this medically contested condition? We limit our discussion to three main themes
that seem to be particularly relevant for contemporary debates about long-term
exhaustion in Western societies: medicalization, normative judgments, and gender
issues.

Cultural and medical constructions
of long-term exhaustion

Definitions of illness as a biological phenomenon are classified as scientific, and
are therefore often seen as more reliable and objective than other forms. By virtue
of being the authority on what illness actually is, the medical system is granted
not only the power to define illness but also the power to create "the social possibilities for acting as sick" (Freidson, 1970, p. 206). The biological dimension,
therefore, becomes dominant in societal definitions. The relation between medical and cultural perceptions of illness, however, is reciprocal: medical definitions
influence cultural definitions at the same time as they influence them.

In the Western world, medical and cultural representations of tiredness and
exhaustion have abounded since at least the time of Hippocrates (fifth century BC),
who believed in a balance of etheric forces essential to the "life body." Variants
of this theory are reflected down the ages, notably in that of the "four humors"
(known from the Hippocratic text corpora and further developed by the Roman
physician Galen, 131–199 AD), which (in one form or another) were widely sub-
scribed to until the late nineteenth century. Within these theories, depletion of the
"life force" or "energies" resulted in, among other things, exhaustion, tiredness,
and fatigue.

By the mid-nineteenth century, around the time that Flaubert's *Emma Bovary*
was published, many changes were taking place in the medical arena. Medicine
was professionalized, and Western nations experienced a "hospital boom" (Abel-
Smith, 1964). The ill of middle-class nineteenth-century societies were usually
nursed in the privacy of their own home, or another place of recuperation: the
"sick-room." Consequently, there is a pervasive presence of the sick-room in the
literature from that period (Herndl, 1993). As Bailin (1994, p.5) observes, "there
is scarcely a Victorian fictional narrative without its ailing protagonist, its depic-
tion of a sojourn in the sickroom." Many novels from this era depict exhausted,

bedridden women who spend much of their time lying on a *chaise longue* or in a bed in a dark, quiet bedroom.[2]

Society more generally was also undergoing huge transitions during this period, particularly the industrial revolution, capitalism, urban living, and a changing role for women. Against this backdrop, cultural representations of tiredness and exhaustion began to shift. In 1869, the American neurologist George Beard proposed a diagnostic category for the condition, namely neurasthenia, describing it as an organic "lack of nerve-force" (1881, pp. 5–6) caused by pathological changes in the "chemical structure" of the central nervous system (1869, p. 218); and sufferers were reassured that the condition was a not a mental illness: "it is a physical, not a mental state" (1881, p. 17).

The potential causes of nervous fatigue were numerous, but were typically considered to be brought about by modern (industrial) life; it was a disease of living too fast (Weir Mitchell, 1871). Believing physical, mental, and reproductive energies to be in competition with each other, an excess or abuse of one was considered to cause depletion or surplus of another (e.g. excessive female intellect or study could cause infertility). Beard derived his theory of neurasthenia from the "brain workers" of the American business class. Thus, in the early days at least, neurasthenia was primarily diagnosed among professional, intellectual, and upper- and middle-class men. By the time *The Yellow Wallpaper* was published in 1892, neurasthenia had been declared a veritable pandemic.

In contemporary Western societies, long-term unexplained exhaustion is medically described with diagnostic labels such as Chronic Fatigue Syndrome (CFS), burnout, and Myalgic Encephalomyelitis (ME). All these labels refer to a medically unexplained, debilitating long-term exhaustion that cannot be directly associated with an organic pathology. These conditions are a site of ongoing controversy, as researchers and patients differ profoundly on the degree to which the cause and course of symptoms may be understood as physical, psychological, or psychosomatic. The most common diagnosis today, ME, was originally presumed to be a viral infectious disease, but was reinterpreted in the 1970s as caused by psychological factors. This change was fused by two English psychiatrists who argued that an outbreak in London (1955) had been an episode of mass hysteria that usually occurred "in populations of segregated females – in girls' schools, convents, and among female factory hands" (McEvedy and Beard, 1970, p. 9). The assumed mechanism is that a lack of coping with stress can cause damage to the nervous system. Patient-led counter-movements began to develop in the late 1980s. However, initially sympathetic media coverage soon became antagonistic as doctors and journalists proposed disparaging explanations related to the personalities of sufferers. The debate has remained polarized ever since (Aronowitz, 1998; de Wolfe, 2009).

The three fictional texts

Madame Bovary (1857) is the French author Gustav Flaubert's debut novel. Flaubert was accused of immorality and had to go through a trial before the over

300-page novel could be published in April 1857. However, the novel quickly became a bestseller, and today it is considered one of the most famous novels of literary realism. *Madame Bovary* has been described as one of the most unforgettable figures in all modern prose fiction (Micale, 1995).

The main character of the novel – Emma Bovary – is the daughter of a wealthy farmer and married in the beginning of the novel to graduate doctor Charles Bovary, who has his practice in rural northern France. Life in the province does not correspond to Emma's expectations and aspirations, and she is disappointed with her husband. A feeling of boredom and longing for something more pulls her into two different, doomed, extramarital relationships. Motherhood does not fulfill Emma's quest for meaning. Finally, Emma allows herself to be led toward complete self-destruction; she acquires arsenic in an apothecary (Homais) and takes her own life. Her husband is devastated and dies shortly afterward; their daughter is left to grow up with relatives and must work in a cotton-spinning mill.

A prolific and activist writer in her time, Charlotte Perkins Gilman's *The Yellow Wallpaper* (1892) has endured as her most well-known work. This short story became a bestseller soon after it was first published in January 1892 in *The New England Magazine*. Gilman herself was diagnosed as neurasthenic, and *The Yellow Wallpaper* was inspired by the treatment of Dr. Silas Weir Mitchell, the doctor who tried to cure her. An important aspect of Gilman´s short story is that she uses "nervous" illness in a deliberately metaphorical and political way, which complicates our reading of her text.

Gilman's short story unfolds entirely in the physical and mental confines of her bedroom. The unnamed protagonist, who is also the narrator, has been brought to the countryside by her husband John (who is a doctor) to recover following a birth with subsequent depression and fatigue (interpreted as both hysteria and neurasthenia, or what we might now identify as postpartum depression). There, she is banished to her bed to undergo a "rest cure." She is forbidden to work, even to take her daily diary notes or write in any way.

During her period of confinement, the protagonist glides slowly into an irrational, parallel universe where her bedroom and the yellow wallpaper play a pivotal metaphorical function. Toward the end of the story, when inaction has transformed depression into psychosis, she imagines herself as a creature that lives in the wallpaper's pattern: her final (symbolic) act is to strip the wallpaper from the room in an effort to free the woman trapped inside – and herself.

The Woman Who Went to Bed for a Year (2012) is the last novel of Sue Townsend, an acclaimed British writer, whose *Adrian Mole* book series went on to sell more copies than any other work of fiction in Britain during the 1980s. Townsend suffered ill health throughout her adult life, and when she wrote her last novel she was confined to a wheelchair with serious sight problems.

In this comic novel we follow our heroine, Eva, a 50-year-old librarian from Leicester and a married mother of two teenagers, who decides to stay in bed for one year the same day as her children move away from home to study at Leeds University. As the novel develops, we (and Eva) learn that her husband has been unfaithful to her for the past eight years. Throughout the novel, there is fierce opposition to Eva withdrawing from the world. At the same time, Eva strives to dispel the theories of her friends, family, and medical professionals that she is suffering from a mental illness ("empty nest syndrome" or a "mental breakdown" of some kind), and indeed, that she is ill at all. During her time in bed, Eva reappraises her entire life – and reflects on the absurdity of domestic life and suburban living. It is through her time in bed that she begins to understand what it means to be free. By the end of the novel, Eva has become a radical figure – a role model for others who aspire to act on their own wishes and desires.

Contextualized analysis and interpretation

Our search for convergence and divergence of sociocultural understandings of tiredness and exhaustion across the three fictional texts revealed several interesting patterns. In the following, we discuss three of the most interesting themes.

Theme 1: Medicalization

Medicalization is a sociocultural process (Illich, 1975) through which a human experience is culturally redefined from an experience to a medical condition. In our case, medicalization implies (1) viewing and describing long-term exhaustion through the use of medical terminology (i.e. diagnosis); (2) using medical explanations to explain its causes; and/or (3) using medical technology to try to cure it (Conrad, 1992). We ask: in what ways and to what extent is long-term fatigue presented in a medicalized manner in the three works of fiction?

Diagnosis and etiology: assigning a label and searching for a cause

Written before Beard's diagnostic labels became widely used, Flaubert does not label Emma Bovary with diagnostic categories like neurasthenia or hysteria, but very occasionally (five times) uses the label "nervous," "nervous complaint," or "nervousness" to characterize her "physical illness" (p. 256). Although Flaubert sometimes uses the term "illness" (nine times), his focus does not rest on a medicalized understanding of her situation. Instead of diagnostic labels Flaubert describes specific ailments Emma suffers from, such as exhaustion, dizziness, weak spells, heart palpitations, and bouts of nerves, which are often (indirectly) portrayed as an expression of her character traits. Flaubert describes her "melancholy tone" (p. 238), "moods" (p. 112), "nervous laugh" (p. 86), "nervous frown" (p. 164), and rapid mood swings: "Some days she chattered on and on with febrile energy; this overexcitement would then suddenly give way to a state of torpor, when she would lie without speaking or stirring" (p. 111). When Emma's illness is viewed through a medical lens, Dr. Bovary's clinical mode of analysis rests on subjectively assessing her symptoms. We occasionally find Dr. Bovary "trying to think what could be the matter with her, imagining it must be a nervous complaint" (p. 165), and, following a bout of vomiting, to "think he recognized the first symptoms of cancer" (p. 186). However, these conjectures are few and far between, and – important to note – *not* conveyed to Emma.

Penned after Beard's taxonomy, Gilman's protagonist is interpreted as having hysteria and neurasthenia as well as postpartum depression, a "temporary nervous depression – a slight hysterical tendency" (p. 5). In the short story, from the doctors' perspectives (both her husband and brother are doctors), her symptoms sometimes take a back seat to the diagnostic labels assigned to them. Nevertheless, the doctors rarely speculate on the underlying cause of the protagonist's illness. Instead, the (potential) cause is subtly presented via the circumstances in which her symptoms arose (postpartum) and the diagnostic labels attached to these symptoms (nervousness, hysteria).

In Townsend's modern-day novel, the evolution of diagnostic categories and the decisive divide between physical and mental health is clearly rendered. Eva's symptoms (exhaustion) are labeled a symptomatic feature of psychological distress, of mental illness. Uncovering the underlying cause of Eva's symptoms is a central theme throughout the novel. Family and friends render the cause apparent from the beginning: "empty-nest syndrome" (p. 4) resulting in a "nervous breakdown" (p. 5). As her mother tells the doctor, "There's nothing much wrong with her, Doctor. It's that syndrome. Empty nest" (p. 70). Likewise, Nurse Spears also informs Eva, "in my opinion, you are having a breakdown of some kind" (p. 285). These interpretations of Eva's actions are common in contemporary medicine: when so-called objective scientific proof of biological pathology is lacking, ailments are easily classified as psychosomatic, and the victims are not only blamed for their illnesses but are also held responsible for sorting it out.

Psyche–soma dualism

Following this theme, we see an increased divide between narrative descriptions and medical interpretations of psyche (mind) and soma (body) across the three fictional works.

In *Madame Bovary*, we find less dualistic psyche and soma imagery than that seen in Townsend's, and, to a lesser extent, Gilman's renderings. We are told on one occasion that Dr. Bovary considers Emma's illness "physical" (p. 256). However, Flaubert rarely distinguishes between physical or psychological etiology when describing Emma's symptoms and experiences. Flaubert depicts Emma's prostration as signifying that "her body and her soul . . . together sought repose after all the turmoil they had known" (p. 186). He explains how "it was her heart that hurt, now her chest, now her head, now her limbs" (p. 186).

In *The Yellow Wallpaper* we see a growing tendency to conceptualize illness in *either* physical *or* mental terms. Gilman's protagonist is direct in her rendering of the doctors' dualistic beliefs, dismissing her "nervous" symptoms as not indicative of "real" (physical) disease: "You see he does not believe I am sick!" (p. 5). Her husband's and brother's doubt that she has a "real" illness seems to rest on assumptions about the inherent weakness of the female character and psyche.

In Townsend's novel we see clear divides (if not rifts) between how psychological and physical aspects of illness are viewed, diagnosed, and treated. One doctor tells Eva that her mother has told him there is nothing wrong with her physically – and he cannot find anything physically wrong either. Another doctor asks the district nurse to "visit a healthy woman who wouldn't get out of bed. . . . The thought of a healthy woman wallowing in bed made her sick, it really did" (p. 113). When the nurse visits Eva in her bed, the latter explains that she is not ill, but the nurse is not convinced:

> Eva said, "Thank you for coming, but I am not ill."
> "Have you undergone medical training?" asked Nurse Spears.
> "No," said Eva, who could see where this exchange was leading. "But I am fully qualified to have an opinion about my own body, I've been studying it for fifty years." . . .
> "I am not ill," she said again.
> "Not physically ill, perhaps, but there must be something wrong with you. It's certainly not *normal* to want to stay in bed for a year, chewing toffees, is it?"
>
> (Townsend, 2012, pp. 115–116)

The medical consultations Eva receives are also divided between a "thorough physical examination" and a "mental health evaluation" (p. 117). An "approved mental health professional" and forcible intervention ("mental health unit," "section four") is recommended (pp. 429–430).

Treatment

In both of our nineteenth-century texts, the clinical focus centers on treating the women's physical symptoms. Emma Bovary is encouraged to seek repose (spending "days in her bed," p. 188) and Gilman's protagonist is banished to bed for "perfect rest" (p. 7). The main treatment for the women is rest, and if mental stimulation is not completely forbidden, it is at the very least discouraged: our protagonist is "absolutely forbidden to "work"" (p. 5) and "Emma was to be prevented from reading novels" (p. 112). A variety of treatments for their symptoms (such as cold water compresses, poultices, valerian and camphor baths, phosphates or phosphites, and tonics) are also administered.

When Gilman wrote her short story "The rest cure" (Weir Mitchell, 1877) was a standard treatment for neurasthenia, at least among women of the middle and upper classes. The cure was based on theories of energy exertion, which proclaimed that rest and recuperation could restore harmony. As Charles Williams wrote in 1848 (p. 10): "the fatigued mind or body is peculiarly prone to suffer from causes of disease . . . and when the body is extremely exhausted, even sleep, which is nature's best restorer, is disturbed."

In contrast, our modern-day protagonist Eva finds that those around her do not understand her need for seclusion and rest. Eva takes the decision to go to bed, and the novel is centered on the attempts of family, friends, and health professionals to get her out of it. The doctor prescribes Eva tablets to minimize her anxiety and recommends mental health assessments. This shift reflects changes in medical treatment beliefs and practices. Current treatments for exhaustion are typically derived from psychological and psychiatric understandings and consist of psychotherapy (e.g. cognitive behavioral therapy) and graded exercise, often coupled with some form of mediation. When Eva refuses to accept these medical (and lay) theories and treatment plans, there are plans afoot to have her institutionalized.

Theme 2: Normative judgments

The moral quality of the main characters' exhaustion in the three narratives is judged very differently, reflecting the associations between illness and behavior prevalent in each cultural moment. Flaubert described Emma Bovary and her ailments mainly in a morally neutral manner, without judging or condemning her in any way, albeit sometimes with ironic references to the bourgeoisie. Via the words of Charles, her husband, her "moods" were provoked by outside influences: "She had moods when she was easily provoked into outrageous behavior" (p. 112). He repeats this non-judgmental view of her in an explicit way several times:

> Why did she fly into these tempers? He blamed everything on her old nervous complaint; and, reproaching himself for confusing physical illness with defects of character, he accused himself of selfishness, and longed to go and take her in his arms.
>
> (Flaubert, 2004[1857], p. 256)

Throughout the novel, Charles demonstrates his devotion several times. During one episode we find that "for forty-three days Charles never left her bedside. He abandoned all his patients; he no longer went to bed" (p. 186). He shows empathy: "Charles wept when he saw her eat her first slice of bread and jam" (ibid.), and understanding: "'You will tire yourself, sweetheart' said Bovary. And, gently urging her into the arbour: 'Sit down on this bench; you'll be alright here'" (ibid.). The only exception to this non-judgmental assessment is a statement from her mother-in-law:

> 'Do you know what your wife really needs?" resumed Madame Bovary senior. "What she needs is hard work, manual labour. If she was obliged to earn her living like so many have to do, she wouldn't suffer from these vapours, which come from all these ideas she fills her head with, and living such an idle life."
>
> (Flaubert, 2004[1857], p. 112)

Emma herself tries to compensate for her ailment through embarking on various extramarital relationships, and spending money on material goods. However, her efforts are in vain. All these bring her are unhappy love affairs and economic bankruptcy. At less than 30 years old she ends her life by taking poison. Still, Flaubert did not present her adultery, material consumption, or eventual suicide as self-imposed, morally improper actions. Madame Bovary's character demonstrates the ways in which the cultural circumstances of bourgeois society (as opposed to individual free will) determined the position of women at that time: the home and the family were status symbols (measured against the rude commercial world), the center of virtue and the cornerstone of an appropriate life for middle- and upper-class women.

In *The Yellow Wallpaper* we see a greater degree of social mistrust of individuals with exhaustion than that seen in *Madame Bovary*. Gilman's protagonist tells the reader, "Nobody would believe what an effort it is to do what little I am able" (p. 8). A growing tendency to blame the (female) victim for their ailment is also reflected in the narrative. The protagonist tells us that her physician-husband holds her responsible for her ailment and for sorting it out: "He says no one but myself can help me out of it, that I must use my will and self-control and not let any silly fancies run away with me" (p. 13).

By contrast, a main theme in Townsend's novel is the lack of understanding and acceptance in society and among people around Eva for her actions. People around her confront her with a mixture of outrage and puzzled disbelief. Her mother reacts with a mix of despair and moral condemnation: "Look at her now! Lolling about in bed like the Queen of Sheba. . . . I didn't bring her up to be a lazy cow" (pp. 101–102), and advises Eva's husband (Brian), "If I were you, I'd starve her out of bed" (p. 154). At the same time, those around Eva explain her actions as an expression of a mental illness. Eva's efforts to combat this understanding of her situation may be interpreted as a cultural critique of this kind of medicalization and psychologicalization of the human condition.

Theme 3: Femininity as a disease: the division between feminine madness and masculine rationality

Which gendered sociocultural norms are expressed in the three fictional works, and how are these embedded in the descriptions of tiredness and exhaustion?

Ideas about women's constitution

Both *Madame Bovary* and *The Yellow Wallpaper* express nineteenth-century views of women as constitutionally weaker than men. At that time, "to be a woman is to be ill" (Michelet, 1853, p. 52), and " every woman is, according to temperament and other circumstances, always more or less an invalid" (Allan, 1869, p. cc). Rest and relaxation were regarded as treatments for tiredness and exhaustion, but were also behaviors expected of women.

In *Madame Bovary, this* view of women is explicitly expressed a number of times: "Women, you know, they get upset over nothing! My wife particularly.

And we'd be wrong to complain about it, because their nervous system is so very much more sensitive than ours" (Monsieur Homais to Charles Bovary, Flaubert, 2004[1857], p. 108). The expressed cultural views on women in *The Woman Who Went to Bed for a Year* are not very different from what we see in the nineteenth-century texts. Although rarely made explicit in the novel, Eva's portrayal bears a strong resemblance to contemporary stereotypes of fatigue as a gendered condition: exhausted, well-educated women with jobs outside their homes are unable to cope with the stress and pressure they impose upon themselves when they fail to respect the limits of their capacity (Lian and Bondevik, 2015).

The myth of female fulfillment

Each work tells a tale of female domestic fulfillment – as wives and mothers – that did not come to fruition, and that leads, one way or another, to the women staying in bed, tired and exhausted. We see in the narratives that the intellectual passions of these women are thwarted by their gender and domestic circumstances. We find that, as a young girl, Emma Bovary "devoured" novels and "spent six months breathing the dust of old lending libraries . . . enthralled by all things historical" (p. 34); the protagonist in *The Yellow Wallpaper* was a keen writer and thinker (as was Gilman); and Eva was a university graduate and had a career as a librarian. However, the women's circumstances, not only during, but leading up to their illness, discourage intellectual activity and pursuits. As modern-day Eva tells us, "I haven't used my brain for so long the poor thing is huddled in a corner waiting to be fed" (Townsend, 2012, p. 41). Moreover, we find that the women's "thinking" (searching for something other than domestic life) may have in some way caused, or contributed to, their exhaustion and unhappiness.

In the late nineteenth-century, the mental labor of "brain workers" was often cited by Beard and others as a cause of nervous disease and exhaustion. This was especially the case for women: "Many women never get over a long and ambitious course of study . . . . . . Many a brilliant student or vigorous athlete has been thus wrecked, perhaps for life – especially among women" (Allbutt and Rolleston, 1905–1911, p. 151). Weir Mitchell's rest cure reflected his patriarchal convictions and general distrust of women, and his seemingly contradictory respect for women's domestic work. Weir Mitchell himself said of neurasthenic women: "She is not fairly up to what nature asks from her as wife and mother" (1871, p. 141). After she had completed her treatment, Weir Mitchell himself gave Gilman the infamous advice to 'Live as domestic a life as possible. Have your child with you all the time. . . . Have but two hours' intellectual life a day. And never touch pen, brush or pencil as long as you live" (Gilman, 1935, p. 96).

One might expect that the theories of the past have no grounds in contemporary thinking. However, similar theories resonate in the present day. In *The Woman Who Went to Bed for a Year*, everyone around Eva immediately assumes that she is suffering from "empty nest syndrome." Her exhaustion and need for solitude and rest are explained by a change in domestic circumstances. Moreover, Eva, like Emma and Gilman's protagonist, is discouraged from "thinking." From her husband's perspective, she has no need:

Eva: "I can't think with you in the house" . . .
Brian: "What have you got to think about?"
Eva: "Everything . . ."
Brian: . . . "I'm the Mensa member. I can do your thinking for you."

(Townsend, 2012, pp.104–105)

Rejection of patriarchy and medical authority

All three women in our fictional texts are married to doctors (medical or academic), whose needs, wants, and desires eclipse their own; and across the works we can see a progressive rejection of medical authority and patriarchy. In our interpretative context, this is shown through the women's fight for the right to free will and self-determination, and their rejection of marital trappings, domestic drudgery, and prescribed medical treatments.

In Flaubert's novel, Emma often seems to comply with Charles's medical recommendations. At points in her illness Emma "refused any kind of treatment" (p. 112); however, few negotiations are present on this front. We also find in Emma a woman who rejects her domestic situation. Following her illness, Emma "just let everything in the house go . . . Emma, always in the past so fastidious and refined, now spent whole days without dressing properly" (p. 59), Later, "she seemed to take no interest in anything beyond her own health" (p. 188), to the point where "She would hardly even bother to give her child a kiss. The dinner wasn't ready, but she didn't care!" (p. 237).

In *The Yellow Wallpaper* the protagonist is confined to the room that functioned as the nursery of the house (the "atrocious nursery," p. 4), which can be read as symbolic of the entrapment of motherhood, marriage, and domesticity. The protagonist often disagrees with the doctors, but rarely explicitly: "Personally, I disagree with their ideas. Personally, I believe that congenial work, with excitement and change, would do me good" (p. 6). She confides to us: "I lie down ever so much now. John says it is good for me. . . . It is a very bad habit, I am convinced, for you see I don't sleep" (p. 16). When she does express disagreement, John invokes his medical (and male) authority: "Can you not trust me as a physician when I tell you so?" (p. 15). It is not until the very end of the story that the protagonist truly defies her husband – and doctor – when she strips the wallpaper to free the woman, her alter-ego, whom she believes is trapped inside. In her own life, Gilman explicitly linked her ailments to male patriarchy and domestic life: her sickness vanished when she was away from her husband and child, and returned as soon as she came home again (Gilman, 1935).

At the beginning of *The Woman Who Went to Bed for a Year*, our modern-day protagonist is also found to be trapped by her gender and domestic circumstances. Before Eva takes to her bed she pours tomato soup all over her most precious chair. She is unhappy in her marriage, and with what her life has become. When her mother declares the diagnosis "empty nest syndrome" Eva objects, and explains that she was "glad to see the back of them" (p. 19) and that she had "been counting the days until they left home from the day the moment they were born! . . . It felt as though I had been taken over by two aliens," she said (p. 70). Eva explicitly expressed her actions as a result of a free choice: "All I wanted to do was go to bed alone and stay there for as long as I liked" (p. 70). Eva also gives up any sense of domestic duty, as her husband Brian says to Alexander, Eva's soon-to-be lover: "Ignore the mess, man, the missus is pulling a sickie!" (p. 86).

Contrary to the nineteenth-century narratives, Eva has no qualms about directly confronting medical authority, rejecting both lay diagnoses and what health professionals tell her. Throughout the novel Eva maintains that she is not ill, and that there is nothing wrong with her. Eva also completely refuses to comply with treatment; the doctor gives her a prescription for a drug that is supposed to minimize her anxiety, which she rips up the minute he leaves the room.

Synthesis of main findings

While looking for similarities and differences across the three works of fiction in relation to our three main themes, we find several interesting patterns. First, we see how representations and understandings of long-term exhaustion have shifted from culturally positioned phenomena (contextualized human experiences) to symptoms that need to be viewed through an individualistic medical and diagnostic lens. This change mirrors the medicalization of long-term fatigue that appeared in the medical system: in the second part of the nineteenth century, long-term exhaustion became defined as a medical condition with the diagnostic label of neurasthenia. With the label and the medical attention, the ailment became medicalized and was thereby made relevant for intervention. We also see how the nineteenth-century perception of exhaustion as a physical disease shifted to a modern-day understanding of (unexplained) exhaustion as a somatic symptom caused by psychological factors. Facets of this medicalization are particularly evident in Townsend's novel. The story about Eva and her self-chosen year in bed is a typically *modern* story with clear traces of our time. The most obvious sign is how people around her seek medical explanations for her actions. Her "action" is explained not as a chosen action (a self-imposed withdrawal from the world) but as an expression – that is, a symptom – of an illness. In contemporary Western societies, there is no other way to make her actions intelligible than via medical theories. Because this illness cannot be seen and validated through medical, technological findings, it is classified as a mental disorder.

Connected to this medicalization, we can trace how normative judgments about exhaustion have changed over time, most notably that in contemporary society people have to fight to legitimatize their symptoms (exhaustion), and their need to rest. Since rest has become increasingly viewed as a morally loaded solution to exhaustion, we see across the narratives how representations of social empathy and understanding of exhaustion have declined over the years, accompanied by an increased tendency to blame the victim. By modern, mainstream medical and cultural standards, it is no longer acceptable to sojourn in the "sick room." Today, tiredness and exhaustion are signs of weakness that must be fought and hidden (Widerberg, 2005). In this cultural context, psychogenic explanations of long-term exhaustion run the risk of stigmatizing the sufferer.

Across all our texts we find that the women's ailments are presented as a "female malady," and the problem lies with the female character and psyche. In all three works, the women's sexual-socioeconomic circumstances are also presented either (subtly or implicitly) as a causal explanation for their illness. Flaubert's and Gilman's texts reflect the nineteenth-century view of woman saying that "to be a woman is to be ill." In Townsend's text we see the silhouette of the upper-class woman of the nineteenth century imposed upon the body of the woman of the twenty-first century, a legacy of failure to cope with the stress of expending her energy both in and out of her home.

By synthesizing these key findings, a core pattern emerges: long-term exhaustion changed from being portrayed as a character trait associated with upper-class women (partly a natural feature and partly a result of their socioeconomic position), to an illness associated with well-educated women working for wages who are unable to cope with the stress and pressure they impose upon themselves when they fail to respect the limits of their capacity. Changes identified through the analysis of the three literary texts are very similar to changes identified in medical constructions of long-term medically unexplained exhaustion. Today, the epidemiology of this condition has been described as reflecting "an excessive risk for educated adult white women," sometimes with "unachievable ambition" and "poor coping skills" (Straus *et al.*, 1988, p. 791). The typical patient is often portrayed with a "female touch" and stereotyped as a well-educated and previously successful middle-class woman with an ambitious and perfectionist personality (Hart and Grace, 2000). This is the energy theory of the 1800s, dressed in modern individualist clothing. Hence, the stigmatizing view of women as particularly receptive to this condition has prevailed but with a major difference: while nineteenth-century women were seen as determined, partly by nature and partly by culture, to be particularly vulnerable, lack of coping is the key element in Townsend's novel. This change reflects the modern neoliberal individualistic perspective on health and illness: through our individual lifestyle choices we our solely responsible for preserving our health and preventing illness. The condition has become more medicalized, but instead of removing blame, as medicalization often does, the ailment is now portrayed in a harmfully judgmental manner.

Notes

1 Medical and fictional representations may be more closely connected than is usually assumed: Steven Heath (1992) has argued that Flaubert used medical textbooks and was inspired by their descriptions of hysteria when he formed the character of Emma and her symptoms, and also that medical textbooks later used Flaubert's descriptions in their definition of hysteria (Heath, 1992; Bondevik, 2007).
2 Among the most famous fictional works are Dumas's *La dame aux camélias* (1848), Flaubert's *Madame Bovary* (1857), Tolstoy's *Anna Karenina* (1873–1877), Bjørnson's *Over Ævne 1* (1883), Ibsen's *The Lady From the Sea* (1888), and Gilman's *The Yellow Wallpaper* (1892).

References

Abel-Smith, B. (1964). *The Hospitals 1800–1948, A Study in Social Administration in England and Wales*. London: Heinemann.

Abrams, P. (1982). *Historical Sociology*. New York: Cornell University Press.

Allan, J.M.G. (1869). On the real differences in the minds of men and women. *Journal of the Anthropological Society of London, 7*, cciv–ccxix.

Allbutt, T.C. and Rolleston, H.D. (1905–1911). Diseases of the brain and mental diseases. In *T.C.* Allbutt and H.D. Rolleston (eds), *A System of Medicine* (Vol. III) (pp. 134–163). London: McMillan and Co.

Antoft, R., Jacobsen, M.H. and Knudsen, L.B. (2010). The poetic imagination – about the relationship between sociology and fiction. In R. Antoft, M.H. Jacobsen, and L.B. Knudsen (eds), *The Poetic Imagination – About the Relationship between Sociology and Fiction* (pp. 13–27). Aalborg: Aalborg University.

Aronowitz, R.A. (1998). *Making Sense of Illness: Science, Society and Disease*. Cambridge: Cambridge University Press.

Bailin, M. (1994). *The Sickroom in Victorian Literature: The Art of Being Ill*. Cambridge: Cambridge University Press.

Beard, G.M. (1869). Neurasthenia, or nervous exhaustion, *The Boston Medical and Surgical Journal, 3*(13), 217–221.

Beard, G.M. (1881). *American Nervousness: Its Causes and Consequences*. New York: Putnam's Sons.

Bjørnson, B. (2012) [1883]. *Over Ævne: Første Stykke, Volume 1*. Denmark: Nabu Press.

Bondevik, H. (2007). *Hysteri i Norge. Et sykdomsportrett* [Hysteria in Norway. A Portrait of a Disease]. Oslo: UNIPUB.

Bourdieu, P. and Ferguson, P.P. (1988). Flaubert's point of view. *Critical Inquiry, 14*(3), 539–562.

Conrad, P. (1992). Medicalization and social control. *Annual Review of Sociology, 18*, 209–232.

de Wolfe, P. (2009). ME: The rise and fall of media sensation. *Medical Sociology Online, 4*(1), 2–13.

Dumas, A. (2008) [1848]. *La dame aux camélias*. Oxford: Oxford University Press.

Flaubert, H.S. (2004) [1857]. *Madame Bovary*. Oxford: Oxford University Press.

Freidson, E. (1970). *The Profession of Medicine. A Study of the Sociology of Applied Knowledge*. Chicago, IL: The University of Chicago Press.

Gilman, C.P. (2016) [1892]. *The Yellow Wallpaper*. Sweden: Wisehouse Classics.

Gilman, C.P. (2011) [1935]. *The Living of Charlotte Perkins Gilman*. Madison: The University of Wisconsin Press.

Hart, B. and Grace, V.M. (2000). Fatigue in chronic fatigue syndrome: A discourse analysis of women's experiential narratives. *Health Care Women International, 21*(3), 187–201.

Hearnshaw, L.S. (1964). *A Short History of British Psychology 1840–1940*. London: Methuen.

Heath, S. (1992). *Flaubert: Madame Bovary*. Cambridge: Cambridge University Press, pp. 53–117.

Herndl, D.P. (1993). *Invalid Women. Figuring Feminine Illness in American Fiction and Culture*. Chapel Hill: The University of North Carolina Press.

Ibsen, H. (2010) [1888]. *The Lady From the Sea*. London: A&C Black.

Illich, I. (1975). The medicalization of life. *Journal of Medical Ethics, 1*, 73–77.

Lian, O. and Bondevik, H. (2015). Medical constructions of long-term exhaustion, past and present. *Sociology of Health and Illness, 37*(6), 920–935.

McEvedy, C.P. and Beard, A.W. (1970). Concept of benign myalgic encephalomyelitis. *British Medical Journal*, *1*(5687), 11–15.

Micale, M.S. (1995). *Approaching Hysteria: Disease and its Interpretation*. Princeton, NJ: Princeton University Press.

Michelet, J. (1858). *L'Amour*. Paris: Calmann-Levy (1898). Cited in L. Jordanova (1989) *Sexual Visions: Images of Gender in Science and Medicine between the Eighteenth and Twentieth Centuries*. Hemel Hempstead: Harvester Wheatsheaf.

Schaffner, A.K. (2016). Exhaustion and the pathologization of modernity. *Journal of Medical Humanities*, *37*, 327–341.

Straus, S.E., Dale, J.K., Wright, R. and Metcalfe, D.D. (1988). Allergy and the chronic fatigue syndrome. *Journal of Allergy and Clinical Immunology*, *81*(5), 791–795.

Thompson, J. (2015). *Jane Austen and Modernization*. New York: Palgrave Macmillan.

Tolstoy, L (2014) [1873–1877]. *Anna Karenina*. Oxford: Oxford University Press.

Townsend, S. (2012). *The woman who went to bed for a year*. London: Penguin Books.

Weir Mitchell, S. (1871). *Wear and Tear: Or, Hints for the Overworked*. Philadelphia, PA: Lippincott Company.

Weir Mitchell, S. (1877). *Fat and Blood, and How to Make Them*. London: J.B. Lippincott & Co.

Widerberg, K. (2005). Embodied gender talks – The gendered discourse of tiredness. In D. Morgan, B. Brandth and E. Kvande (eds), *Gender, Bodies and Work* (pp. 101–112). Hampshire: Ashgate.

Williams, C.J.B. (1848). *Principles of Medicine, Comprising General Pathology and Therapeutics, and a Brief General View of Etiology, Nosology, Semiology, Diagnosis, Prognosis and Hygienics*. London: Churchill.

9 The brute within

Psychosomatic illness and
narrative in *The Sopranos*

Camelia Raghinaru

Psychosomatic illness as rhetoric is present in theories of psychosomasis that reveal the patient as one who suffers from a performative illness. Judy Segal (2008) notes that the "iteration of a circulating narrative of disease" (p. 71) subjects the patient to a process of "internal rhetoric" (p. 80) modeled on the symptoms of disease. Catherine Belling (2012) presents it as a postmodern condition of uncertainty and doubt, which demands careful attention paid to language, in the absence of medical proof, as well as to the disillusionment that comes with the realization of the limitations of medical and scientific certainty. The absence of a determined and identifiable medical threat makes the condition even more pervasive and terrifying for the patient, at the same time as it imbues it with irony and melodrama. In ways of offering a definition of psychosomatic illness for this argument, I will employ Catherine Belling's definition of somatization as "the displacement of psychological, emotional conflicts onto the body such that they are experienced as somatic symptoms. In cases diagnosed as somatization, the patient's body is understood as the proxy for a mental disorder" (p. 16).

The popular TV series *The Sopranos* (1999–2007) features its protagonist, Tony Soprano, as one such patient who deals with psychosomatic symptoms (i.e. successive fainting spells and unexplained panic attacks) that occur, as we come to understand, concomitantly with Tony's exposure to pressures in his family and business life. These he seeks to address through psychoanalytical treatment. The series introduces Tony at the height of his powerful, yet polarized, position as family man and mobster challenged by rivals and problems stemming from his Mafia dealings, but also as an existential character who questions his position in the narrative of the American Dream. A manipulative and duplicitous character, Tony's narrative in Dr. Melfi's office obscures one dimension of his mobster reality while revealing another: the disappointment and existential crisis over having arrived too late into the American narrative of opportunistic heroic conquest, where an immigrant could start a new beginning in a "physical landscape [of vast panoramic frontiers] with the promise of economic opportunity" (as Teena Gabrielson (2009, par. 4) puts it). The metanarrative of "the sun setting over the empire" governs Tony's confessional narrative and explains, to some extent, his depression and anxiety to maintain and increase both his power as the head of a Mafia group and the economic security of his family. Insofar as the feeling is common to many Americans (as Dr. Melfi observes in response), Tony's panic attacks acquire a universality that transcends his unlikely Mafioso circumstances into a universal "expression of racial anxiety, in which he comes unconsciously to recognize the disavowed historicity of his own whiteness" (Kocela, 2005, p. 22).

Christopher Kocela's insight into the nature of Tony's panic attacks brings into discussion two competing types of rhetoric which Tony employs to simultane- ously justify and incriminate himself as a mobster: on the one hand, he struggles to process the complications derived from his racialized position as an Italian- American in a multiracial America of uncertain economic prospects; on the other hand, he uses this very marginalized position to justify his illegitimate dealings, by claiming that he is automatically barred from a legitimate position of power by nature of his schismatic ethnic and anxiety-ridden middle-class position (built on the uncertain foundation of a childhood governed by an abusive bipolar mother and murderously aggressive mobster father). Tony uses:

> the antitheses of his reality as an opportunity to exert more power in force- ful actions. He, therefore, does not deconstruct his own stereotype by dis- mantling mob constructs as one would normally expect from psychoanalytic therapy, but uses therapy to foster a magic of power that consolidates his personal worldview.
>
> (Ricci, 2014, p. 186)

And yet, Tony struggles with his narrative and often feels himself "slipping through the crevices of confessional language" (Ricci, 2014, p. 186), especially in moments when he is trapped in his own duplicity and when "the malevolent image of his neurotic disorder strikes notes too strident to bear" (Ricci, 2014, p. 186). In those instances the narrative of confession performs in ways that are mutually exclusive: on the one hand, Tony is the "modern echo of a primitive warrior, an alpha male" (Ricci, 2014, p. 187), or what he prefers to call the Gary Cooper type, silent, strong, self-assured, and unwavering in his pursuit; on the other, the help- less, whiny victim presupposed by the therapeutic discourse, who has to look for, and acknowledge, the chinks in his armor, resentfully turning against his thera- pist. Tony Soprano fits the description of the psychosomatic patient as victim of unpredictable patterns of life in the modern city: "Violently ruthless, willfully delusional, suffering from bipolar depression, his meteoric rise in the underworld could well mirror an eventual precipitous demonic fall" (Ricci, 2014, p. 165).

In Tony Soprano's case, a psychoanalytical approach is useful to elucidate the connection between narrative, rhetoric and psychosomatic illness, given my argument that psychosomasis is a rhetorical illness and narrative its performa- tive medium. However, narrative is also extraneous to psychosomasis. Psycho- somasis is a type of unconscious, unthought, and psychoanalysis can access it at the level of memories and images. The root cause of Tony's psychosomasis is a violent image of his father chopping off a delinquent debtor's thumb. Narra- tive, particularly as evinced during the therapeutic talk cure, consists of a perfor- mance of psychosomatic illness – an attempt to perform as presence that which is forever obscure and unmediated. Performance is pushing beyond the surface into an inaccessible space. The psychoanalytical narrative challenges standard medical discourse precisely because it is a performance that resists normativity. In this regard, narrative is transgressive because it dissipates the authority of medical discourse. Moreover, in a 1962/1963 seminar, Lacan suggests that anxiety becomes a problem for the Subject whose structure of the Symbolic–Imaginary (i.e. the framework that defines his position in the world) is shattered by a breakthrough of the surplus of the Real (Strubbe and Vanheule, 2014, p. 244). The Real, with psychosomatic illness as its marker, is akin to the *Unheimlich*, the uncanny – this is the name for "everything that ought to have remained . . . secret and hidden but has come to light" (Strubbe and Vanheoule, 2014, p. 244). "This evokes helplessness, to which the experience of panic bears witness" (Strubbe and Vanheule, 2014, p. 244). The confrontation with excess triggers anxiety, and "the body, so to speak, spirals into a state of uproar" (Strubbe and Vanheule, 2014, p. 246) – an evocative image for psychosomasis as narrative that spirals out of control.

Franco Ricci (2014) interprets Tony Soprano's panic attacks as a fall out of language, where the stifling of speech and the fall into silence interrupt and displace Tony's meaning. Under the influence of the attack, and as a silenced, comatose, unconscious body, Tony "is similar to an iconic object because his whole function as a text is suspended" (p. 184). I place Tony's psychosomatic illness (i.e. his panic-induced fainting spells) at the intersection between body (the iconic mobster, albeit weakened and vulnerable) and mind (the split self struggling to construct a stable identity in order to prevent the fainting spells from undermining his public image). His psychosomatic symptoms "open an incidental space of uncontrollable discourse" (p. 185) in his tough mobster façade. "These attacks are micro-discourses that interrupt the normal paradigmatic strata of mob syntagma" (p. 184). Despite his code of the silent, strong, hardboiled gangster, Tony uses language as protection against the splitting of the self. Rhetoric binds together the broken, disparate pieces of the many roles he plays in daily life. In fact, Catherine Belling (2012) identifies psychosomasis as "a problem of knowing, telling, and anxious imagining" (p. 1), a condition of knowledge and doubt, when an individual is confronted with "the stresses of irreconcilable conflict" (p. 2).

The narrative outpouring during his therapy sessions with Dr. Melfi is meant to deceive his therapist and delude Tony himself with the illusion that he can mesh together the irreconcilable scripts of father, suburbanite neighbor, respectable community member, and underground gangster. The panic attacks constitute his only moments of lucidity, as it were, where the narrative of deceit is interrupted and flashes of the Real break through. In terms of unconscious truth, Tony's panic attacks stand on a par with his dreams, coma, or his peyote-induced revelation, when again, the Real impinges upon the Symbolic. His psychosomatic attacks are literally a way for the psyche to break out of the prison of language and take control of the body in a way that would alert Tony to the reality of his existence. Ironically, Tony's therapy sessions ultimately perfect his ability to lie, and it is after five years of therapy that Tony is able to solidify his remorseless mobster self and get rid of any pangs of consciousness that had been bothering him before the therapy. If the panic attacks indicate a struggle in Tony's consciousness, some lucidity and humanity struggling to coexist in tension with the brute within, at the end of the therapy session Tony is cured of his attacks, and also of the little bit of humanity that was causing the rift. Perhaps the success and failure of Dr. Melfi's approach with Tony is that she recognizes that, as Belling (2012) puts it, Tony's psychosomatic condition has to be approached not from a position of mastery (medical, moral, or otherwise), but from a position of a gap in mastery (p. 2).

During his sessions with Dr. Melfi, Tony's narrative gives shape to the form-lessness of his anxiety, which is otherwise passive and in need of a linguistic shape. Narrative is also a way of creating and maintaining the lone ranger ideal that is Tony's norm of masculinity, extinct in modern life, but surviving in the original tale of the frontier myth that "offers a means for deploying the physical environment materially and symbolically to mediate deep contemporary tensions between economic security and domestic felicity" (Gabrielson, 2009, par. 2). Narrative connects past to present: it is a function of survival for the melancholic, a function of rage, but it is like an open secret: it conceals as much as it shows. Narrative gives meaning, but it also bridges the irrationality of psychosomasis to rational narrative – unmasking but also concealing; it is a form of indifference, but also of deferral. It controls and manages psychosomasis through talk therapy in order to give form to and shape anxiety, but it is a way to imagine the unimagina-ble and thus to get a handle on it. There are traces of psychosomasis in narrative, yet narrative cannot fully capture it. Narrative transforms psychosomasis from pre-language to language by embedding it in language.

Psychosomatic illness is, therefore, performative: it exempts the ill person from certain responsibilities, while it obligates him or her to participate in oth-ers. Tony is able to divert some of the blame for his own actions to the parental figures of his childhood. He complains that he was not supported by his par-ents, in order to excuse his own poor parenting skills, particularly in relation to Anthony Junior. Talking to a therapist is a dangerous occupation in itself for a mobster. However, Tony feels compelled to engage in therapy in order to deal with his anxiety attacks. In the television series, talking to a psychiatrist is asso-ciated with the Rico statutes and mobsters ratting on each other to avoid going to prison. The code of silence, the *omerta*, is a value of the highest rank, to the point that engaging in unsanctioned talking can be more dangerous than a shooting. Moreover, depression also exempts Tony, at least temporarily, from most of his obligations. Christopher observes in a conversation with Silvio, one of Tony's capos, that Tony is sleeping all the time and not taking care of himself, while Carmella notes that this is abnormal even for her husband. Ultimately, Tony feels exempted from life itself: "This shit – I don't feel nothin'. Nothin'. Dead. Empty" (I. 12. "Isabella"). As a consequence, he simply checks out and moves into an idyllic vision of Isabella. The fantasy of Isabella connects to Tony's fear of castration and of the overbearing mother – fears he would never admit to himself but has to entertain in the course of therapy. This triggers a guilt com-plex of the ungrateful son. The ultimate performative act lies in the contradic-tion between Tony's jovial, powerful, confident social mask and the downward spiraling motion of his inner self: "I have to be the sad clown. Laughing on the outside, crying on the inside" (I. 1. "The Sopranos").

In the late 1970s psychosomatic disorders were thought to result from "chronic tension on the autonomic nervous system caused by inappropriately or inadequately expressed emotions" (Malkina-Pikh and Pikh, 2012, p. 206), but also from post-traumatic stress. Consequently, the body's reaction to stress has been associated with anxiety disorders such as post-traumatic stress disorder, panic disorder, generalized anxiety disorder, social anxiety disorder, obsessive compulsive disorder, and sleep disturbances (Malkina-Pikh and Pikh, 2012, p. 206). Yet, it is the argument from uniqueness that makes the psychosomatic patient a special patient (Segal, 2008, p. 81). He is the patient who is sick like no other, though that uniqueness stands in tension with the physician's rhetoric of the generic, textbook case, rather than the idiosyncratic. The patient is in essence in perpetual dialogue, first of all with the self (Segal, 2008, p. 82), trying to persuade with tenacity and anxiety. Psychosomasis is a rhetorical disease, and the patient is a performer: "seeker, calculator, claimant, and persuader of an intolerable ambiguity" (Segal, 2008, p. 83). The therapeutic dialogue seeks to unearth the roots of the illness, which in Tony's case go back to childhood incidents in which he witnesses his emotionally dysfunctional mother threatening to suffocate her children and his brutal, murderous father exacting bloody revenge from delinquent debtors. In therapy, as an adult inhabiting his father's place and mitigating his mother's murderous intentions toward him, Tony is reluctant to work through feelings he would rather leave unexplored. However, as Shoshana Felman (1989) points out, the psychoanalytic encounter does not deal with the patient's passion for self-knowledge, but with his or her passion for ignorance and the "desire to ignore" (p. 79) the revelatory facts about the self. Rather, this is not just resistance to facts, but resistance to one's own involvement in the facts. We see this resistance in Tony's refusal to accept his ethical involvement in his own trauma, which marks him as a type of melancholic subject.

Dr. Jennifer Melfi's task is to channel Tony's self-beratement into a narrative that reveals the precise place where Tony resists interpretation – and that has to do with his mother, of course, but also with his conspiracy to protect the mother so that he can continue to perpetuate violence. Felman (1989) capitalizes on the importance of resistance to knowledge as a dynamic act of negation. Resistance to knowledge is equated with a type of ignorance that is akin to forgetfulness, repression, and "the imperative to exclude from consciousness, not to admit to knowledge" (p. 79). Felman writes: "Ignorance is thus no longer simply opposed to knowledge: it is itself a radical condition, an integral part of the very structure of knowledge" (p. 78). "Dialogue is thus the radical condition of learning and of knowledge, the analytically constitutive condition through which ignorance becomes structurally informative; knowledge is essentially, irreducibly dialogic" (p. 83). The analyst alone is not a master of knowledge, because knowledge is "always in the Other" (p. 83) and it is dynamic: "It is not contained by any individual but comes about out of the mutual apprenticeship between two partially unconscious speeches that both say more than they know" (p. 83).

Tony's dialogical relationship with Dr. Melfi leads to Tony's acknowledgment of his mother as a *strega* figure: a castrating, infanticidal force that stands behind Tony's self-destructive impulses and the recent murder attempt commissioned by Junior Soprano in conspiracy with Livia Soprano. Tony's ignorance regarding his mother's motives is willed, and he hangs onto it desperately, violently attacking Dr. Melfi verbally and threatening to assault her physically when she forces the recognition. Immediately before this recognition, two maternal visions pair up in Tony's psyche: one of rusticity, simplicity, and innocence in Avellino, where Isabella appears clad in white, as a new mother cradling a new baby to her breast protectively and caressing it tenderly. (The baby, Dr. Melfi points out, is Tony's fantasy of himself under the protective care of a tender mother.) The other image is that of his own mother, Livia, invoking images of infanticide in various guises: from mentions of mothers throwing their babies out of the window to a conversation between Carmella and Livia regarding Livia's "textbook manipulation" (I. 11. "Nobody Knows Anything") power with which she controls Tony; to a conversation between Livia and her husband which Tony witnesses as a child when Livia threatens to annihilate the children; to yet another conversation between Livia and Junior, where Livia confesses she'd rather see her son dead than the "lobotomized" (I. 12. Isabella") version of the depressed Tony.

According to Jean White (2006), Jacques Lacan links psychosomatic illness to a type of "'suppletion' of a psychotic structure" (p. 113) through which "physical illness might develop as a response to the threat of change or disruption of the organization" (p. 113). White further connects this disruptive threat to the maternal factor:

> The "desomatization" of psyche depends on the introjection of a benign and soothing maternal environment which can contain and process primitive affect. When this is disturbed for some reason, the person may function in a psychosomatic fashion in adult life.
>
> (White, 2006, p. 114)

As Dr. Melfi points out, Livia Soprano and her borderline-type personality is the cause of the disruption in the maternal environment. White writes that borderline states are "fragment forms of narcissism and [stand] between psychosis and neurosis" (p. 115). These people are vulnerable to psychotic breakdowns, and Tony has been on the receiving end of veiled and not-so-veiled threats from his mother. But Tony's complicated relationship with his mother is indicative of a larger problem in the brotherhood of the mafia. In "the remnants of a maternal presence that has been dismissed, marginalized, or recontextualized into an easily digestible masculine context" (Ricci, 2014, p. 143), the feminine space is exploited, dishonored, easily replaceable, and subject to a type of domination that reinforces the phallocentric structure of power of the mob. "Within this masculine mob narrative, the mother–son bond is a reified, sanctified, archetypal herald to be celebrated and supported at all costs" (Ricci, 2014, p. 146). The principle of masculine power is threatened when it encounters its feminine counterpart. This is visible in the relationship between Ralphie, the mobster, and Tracee, his stripper girlfriend, whom he impregnates and mocks for her domestic dreams of stability. Maternity is relegated to a cultural script that is clearly separated from that of the "whore," and this division reinforces the binary upon which the family romance is constructed. Accordingly, "the material spaces of home and strip club do not correspond with the cultural spaces – the ideologies of gender, class, and sexuality – typically attributed to them" (Johnson, 2007, p. 275). As a club worker turned unwed mother, Tracee's claim on Ralphie undercuts his macho act and also reveals Ralphie's ethnic and class-related vulnerability as an Italian-American of little education and blue-collar background, whose status as a "made man" is undermined by his inability to earn for his bosses. Merri Lisa Johnson links women's vulnerability, maternal or otherwise, to a:

> hypermasculine system in which many men are made to feel vulnerable and feminized. Ralphie brutalizes Tracee because she undermines his masculinity in front of his peers. His insecure class status makes it feel imperative to him to protect his masculinity, and his violence against her is a manifestation of this class anxiety at least as much as it is an exercise of patriarchal power.
>
> (Johnson, 2007, p. 284)

Adriana, another victim caught in the victimizing binary of the good girl/bad girl, also suffers from a psychosomatic illness (i.e. ulcerative colitis triggered by her secretive cooperation with the Feds), and thus proves a direct threat to Tony, Christopher, and the "family" at large. In fact, so is any woman with which any of the mobsters have a significant relationship. For instance, Junior Corrado's lover, Roberta, who exposes his "weakness" from the point of view of acceptable macho performance – his penchant for oral sex – is immediately discarded. Women are mere cover-ups and means of detachment, or foils for the men's egos (Ricci, 2014, p. 150). Masculinity is fragile in the show, and it seems trapped, in one way or another, between the hoodlum father and the destructive bipolar mother, much to the psychological detriment of the sons who end up rationalizing violence "as a means of settling accounts and of doing what's right according to the relived memories of [the fathers]" (Ricci, 2014, p. 126). Between the father's mobster legacy as the kiss of death in one way, and the mother's petrifying Medusa stare in another, these sons exhibit a split masculine self, seemingly robust and indestructible on the exterior, and vulnerable, fragile, and insecure on the interior. The ironic treatment of the nuclear family romance reflects a "generalized anxiety over a decline in morality across the generations, especially in the context of socio-economic upward mobility" (Hipsky, 2006, par. 25). Thus, Tony, the epitome of the lost son, "vigorously disassociates himself from what he perceives to be his feminine and plaguing inner nature, and projects his troubled self-repulsion onto the outside world" (Ricci, 2014, p. 129). He also projects, I might add, the trouble within his psyche upon his body in yet another visual and concrete reiteration of the trouble within.

Tony's trouble is not just rooted in his childhood past, but also in his illicit present. As Glenn Strubbe and Stijn Vanheule (2014) point out, "Freud located the cause of actual neuroses [associated here with panic disorder, anxiety neuroses, neurasthenia, and hypochondria] at the level of the drive and connected them to problems in the patient's present-day life, rather than in a repressed event or constellation of events from the past" (p. 238). Freud considered that panic disorder reflected an "immediate 'automatic' or 'traumatic' form of anxiety, which in itself is meaningless, and it is for precisely this reason that it overwhelms the subject" (p. 238). According to Strubbe and Vanheule (2014), Lacan stressed that the experience of being overwhelmed was intrinsic to panic: "a so-called Real element invades consciousness and creates a sudden experience of helplessness" (p. 240). A tired Tony confronts his many-faceted self in therapy, only to be confronted in turn with the "vulnerable underbelly of his false self" (Ricci, 2014, p. 80), the feeling of being caught in-between, of dealing with the issue of lack, the hyphenation of his Italian-Americanness, and his own self-consciousness toward it. The series comments on the false identity of the Italian-American perpetuated by the media in order to instill fear and suspicion as well as to manipulate images "to foster empathy, familiarity, and trust" (Ricci, 2014, p. 81). The Sopranos are "upstart misfits" (Ricci, 2014, p. 85), and their identity oscillates between insularity and the desire for cohesion with the social fabric of society: "On the one hand, the deprecating confidence of a singular national identity is undermined, replaced by an overarching individuality that craves success at any cost" (Ricci, 2014, p. 85).

What Tony, his world, and psychosomatic illness all have in common is an element of excess, which Lacan qualified as the Real that overwhelms the ego trapped in the Symbolic. Transcending a typical medical diagnosis, psychosomatic illness is surplus, excess of the self, since too much awareness stemming from an encounter with the Real unmediated by the Symbolic overpowers the mind and spills over into the body, the repressed returning as somatic symptoms. Psychosomatic illness is the excess that arises after somatic and mental illness have been taken into account. Tony is a voracious consumer – of food, commodities, sex, and even violence. Tony is at the mercy of his own excess of self – the beast within. Johnny Cash's song concludes the pilot episodes on the same note: "The beast in me/is caged by frail and fragile barns/restless by day and by night/rants and rages and at the stars/and God help the beast in me." The song alludes to the violence in the show, but also to the symbolic beast that dominates Tony – his depression and his anxiety – the things he cannot control that control him. This surplus of self belongs to the same category as the Kantian sublime. Tony partakes in his excess even as it crushes him down. There is an aporia, a failure in his illusion of power, because, in the end, he is at the mercy of anyone who wants to take a shot at him: paid mercenaries from the outside, and his own panic from within. That one can seem all powerful, to make life-and-death decisions on the fates of others, but ultimately not to be able to control one's own fate is what leads Tony to wonder obsessively, "Who am I?" This question itself is a type of surplus, since it carries with it "a certain inaccessible Real component, which always escapes the subject" (Strubbe and Vanheule, 2014, p. 243).

Tony's anxiety is triggered by the realization that power is a fiction and that there is a vacuum at its core, both on the micro-scale of the mob business and on the macro-scale of the universe. The universe will collapse, eradicate remnants of life, and end in the disintegration of matter. The existential meaninglessness of life triggers both Tony's and Anthony Junior's panic attacks – the fact that they have no real control over their reality; that the one thing that is absolutely necessary is that nothing is necessary. That everything is contingent is the burden with which Tony has to come to terms. He does so during his peyote-induced delirium, when he finds a type of Nietzschean transcendence beyond good and evil.

Tony and Dr. Melfi have in common the thrill of the encounter with the exposed Real, of peeking beyond the veil of illusion that blinds the "happy whistler." Alex Schulman (2010) argues that what motivates Tony's existential angst is, more than anything, fear of boredom, as a peculiar modern condition. To avoid boredom, Tony has to create his own moments of transcendence, even if that is achieved through addictive or compulsive behaviors (p. 36). This is the sublime of the twentieth-century American cowboy. It is no longer nature's excess that crushes one, but rather the excess of consumerism, unmediated violence, pornography, and sex. It is the suppuration of the self wounded by the Real – the awesome terribleness of postmodern life at the outskirts of legality. And yet, our capacity to imagine our own annihilation gives us the capacity to transcend it. This is the place where Tony gains the most awareness, but also the source of his panic. His fainting spells speak for his silent, horror-filled moments of lucidity and self-awareness and for his "inner self-loathing" (Ricci, 2014, p. 172).

> Since speech is stifled, he no longer produces meaning but is displaced, fixed in spatialized temporality, unable to impose narrative signification. The series arises from his attempts to verbalize the root causes of this trauma, a predicament that he attributes to a sense of dread and existential malaise.
>
> (Ricci, 2014, p. 184)

Angst frustrates Tony's relationship with the social other, and this makes itself manifest in his impossibility to speak of his loss. This impossibility converts, paradoxically, into the incessant and "insistent communicativeness" which in the melancholic amounts to masochistic pleasure derived from "self-exposure" (Butler, 1997, p. 186). The resulting narrative is the only way to imagine psychosomasis, though psychosomasis resists narrative. Narrative is a window into the inner violence wrecked by psychosomasis, rather than a mirror that provides representation and recognition. But at the same time, narrative does a kind of violence to psychosomasis, because narrative consumes and feeds off of psychsomasis as its object. Narrative is about meaning-making, whereas psychosomasis is about the unthought. Narrative's only power is the power of its appearance. It is predicated upon this failure. Its power is dispersed and fragmented. Its power is reflective – hence the danger of fetishization of narrative/language/talk cure. It fails to "cure" Tony. It makes him into a better gangster because it gives him the rationalization and instrumentalization he needs to justify violence. Narrative links inner to outer violence. It is purely subversive.

There is another contradiction at play, however: both protagonists, Tony Soprano and Jennifer Melfi, swing between self-fulfillment and self-destruction (Ricci, 2014, p. 194). "The result is a homogenous unity where underlying personal tension and pathologically morbid structures" (Ricci, 2014, p. 190) working together to bring the end of the series to a type of recognition for both characters. Dr. Melfi finally realizes that therapy for criminals is futile or harmful, because "Tony uses therapy to foster a magic of power that consolidates his personal world view" (Ricci, 2014, p. 186). Tony conquers his qualms and contradictions and resolves to accept with serenity, rather than struggle, his brutal, violent, "tiger" side (a reference to the feline tattooed on his broad shoulders). We are given to understand that his underlying psychosomatic illness, initially triggered by his schizophrenic split between good and evil, his moral struggle, is now healed:

> From the view point of the narrative, self-understanding is the healing fiction that permits him to leave behind acts of linear time and construct new acts of the imagination. . . . The pain of finding a comfortable and sustainable mimesis . . . of his divided self, the dilemma of facing his morally bereft choices, have come to a head and have been resolved.
>
> (Ricci, 2014, p. 188)

Tony's dreams tend to reveal to him the truth about others (as with Pussy Bonpensiero's betrayal) or the truth about himself. His therapy session dream following Christopher's death reveals the union of the two conflicting sides: the convincing liar and the cynical truth-teller. In the dream he switches from one to the other seamlessly, as he convincingly tells Dr. Melfi both that he is pained to see Christopher die in his arms and that Christopher was draining him emotionally. During Tony's next therapy session with Dr. Melfi the dream becomes reality, and Tony voices his relief again, congratulating himself on account of two murders: Christopher's and Adriana's. The clearest proof of the reverse movement in Tony's psychology is his transformation from the "sad clown" to the pretense of sadness that masks his inner relief: "I gotta sit there. . . . And I gotta have the long face and the sighing and the platitudes" (VI. 18. "Kennedy and Heidi").

The ultimate victim of the show is Adriana La Cerva, who fails to receive protection from Christopher, Tony, and the FBI, and is unceremoniously executed for her reluctant betrayal of the mob family. Torn between her allegiance to Christopher, Tony, and the mob, and her desire to get away from the world of crime and restart her life with Christopher under the witness protection program, she carries secrets that undermine her body and soul. Salvatore "Pussy" Bonpensiero falls into the same category, as he suffers from severe, debilitating back pain triggered by the stress of carrying a deadly secret – the betrayal of the mob family to the Feds. Both characters are ultimately killed by the mob because, unlike Tony, they are unable to resolve their tension satisfactorily one way or another before they are caught. Both characters suffer from somatic symptoms as a consequence of emotional and psychological estrangement from their strongest ties: those with the mob (includ-ing his wife and kids, for Pussy, and with her mother, for Adriana), in addition to the stress of carrying a secret. However, Adriana occupies an exclusive place in her extreme marginalization as the abject female gang member, whose main func-tion is to render the more visible and the more pathetic the death of her masculine counterpart Christopher. Overly sexualized, racialized, and marginalized in her complete dependency on her gangster boyfriend, Adriana's disappearance forces the encounter with Death as the unresolved surplus in the series. Hers is an ideo-logical sacrifice. She represents an inverted celebration of triumphant masculinity in a brave-new-world urban landscape in which only men can exist beyond good and evil. Women are punished both for transgressing the boundaries of law, moral-ity, and proper sexuality, and also for attempting to domesticate their free-spirited lawless lovers and return them to the sphere of legality, civility, and domesticity. As a mark of vulnerability in Christopher's life – his only connection to romance, humanity, and goodness – Adriana's execution is inevitable. Hers is a substitution-ary sacrifice. She is killed so that Christopher and Tony can continue their illegal operations. If the male gangsters emerge as strangely appealing in their capacity to balance acts of violence and acts of honesty, female characters like Adriana, Carmella, and the other *goomahs* are pathetic in their abject dependence and facile elimination.

Estrangement, intricate ties of human relationships, and psychosomatic illness are connected in the work of Anthony Vidler (1994). Metropolises as centers of agglomeration (such as New Jersey and New York in the series) are associated with phobias beyond neurasthenia: agoraphobia, claustrophobia, monophobia (fear of solitude and isolation), fear of touching, and other types of spatial fear (p. 19). These phobias fall into the general category of "estrangement" named by sociologists, including Georg Simmel, as a central metaphor for life in the city (p. 19). Simmel argued this had to do with the urban tension between too close an identification with things and at the same time too great a remove from them (quoted in Vidler, 1994, p. 20). The theory of estrangement is tied to the space of the city and the place and role of individuals within it (p. 20). Gabrielson (2009) argues that dramas that question meaning in America take place in the:

> contemporary geo-political context of globalization and advanced capital-ism . . . [and] convey anxiety rather than optimism by emphasizing confine-ment, constraint, and a suffocating sameness in the environs of suburbia. These physical environs then underscore the psychological dislocation from which all characters suffer.
>
> (Gabrielson, 2009, par. 56)

Tony's panic attacks are such an example. Simmel talks about the psychological content derived from the "empty space" between individuals and the way it is filled with the constant ebb and flow of stimuli. Social relations are distanced, alienated, and depersonalized, at a vast remove from the intimate, slower, more habitual rhythms of the small town or rural existence (quoted in Vidler, 1994, p. 21). The adventurer or the stranger are typical personae of this type of cultural life. The stranger is not a wanderer who comes today and goes tomorrow, but the immigrant type, a fixed persona who comes today and stays tomorrow, though never quite belonging (p. 22). "In the stranger are organized the unity of nearness and remoteness of every human relation" (Simmel quoted in Vidler, 1994, p. 22). The stranger is thus modeled on Freud's uncanny. A more concrete materialization of the stranger is that of the vagabond, the *flaneur*, "who alone, criminal and exiled, possessed the marginal vision that transgressed boundaries and turned them into thresholds" (p. 25). Doctor Charcot, who was examining mental diseases in the nineteenth century, identified vagabonds and workers as suffering from attacks of hysteria or epileptic amnesia and periodic loss of memory (p. 26). The urban labyrinth retains something of the nomadic terror of wandering:

> Viewed through these lenses, the urban street regained something of the original terror route. Where the original road carried with it the "terrors of wandering," embedded in the mythical unconsciousness of the wandering tribes, the street engenders a new form of terror, that of the boredom inspired by the "monotonous ribbon of asphalt."
>
> (Vidler, 1994, p. 27)

The modern self is crushed at the intersection of technology, science, bureaucracy, and ideology (Killen, 2006, p. 45). Out of this mix emerges the neurasthenic, "who experiences this conflict with particular intensity" (Killen, 2006, p. 45). His split consciousness mediates between mind and emotions against the backdrop of big city life. This makes neurasthenia an "exemplary condition of modern civilization" (Killen, 2006, p. 47). Martin Hipsky (2006) notes that an unspecified, generalized threat heightened by anxiety and vulnerability characterizes the series. He connects it to the "global paranoia" (par. 3) of capitalism in the metropolis, and specifically to the "nationally mediated experience of the American middle classes, within the milieu of post-Cold War" (par. 33), when a mix of domestic anxieties cross over racial and class structures to amount to rising apprehensions about the future of the next generation. This obsession with the nature of family (both in the domestic and Mafia sense) is at the core of Tony's anxiety, as he makes it his life's purpose to ensure the continuity of his children's economic and class privilege with his project of upward mobility. Yet, due to his morally ambiguous position as *pater familias*, he does so unsuccessfully, because, as Hispky notes, "this authoritative patriarch may represent the fantasy protector of the fragile, vulnerable domestic sphere [as in Dr. Melfi's vengeance fantasy against her rapist, where Tony takes the role of protector and vigilante], but he can also be its greatest threat [as a sociopath who is aware of the kind of example he sets for his children, both of whom follow in his footsteps as young adults]" (par. 38). Tony's illness, therefore, is less about resolving a series of unexplained panic attacks and more about coming to terms with the moral and psychological conflicts inherent in his position. His therapy is not about a cure, but about his acceptance of "the fundamental inadequacies of self-conscious life in modern civilization" (Schulman, 2010, p. 24).

References

Belling, Catherine. (2012). *A Condition of Doubt: The Meaning of Hypochondria*. Oxford: Oxford University Press.

Butler, Judith. (1997). *The Psychic Life of Power: Theories in Subjection*. Stanford, CA: Stanford University Press.

Chase, David (Producer). (1999–2007). *The Sopranos* [Television series]. New York: HBO Home Video.

Felman, Shoshana. (1989). *Jacques Lacan and the Adventure of Insight: Psychoanalysis in Contemporary Culture*. Cambridge, MA: Harvard University Press.

Gabrielson, Teena. (2009). "The end of new beginnings: Nature and the American Dream in *The Sopranos*, *Weeds,* and *Lost*." *Theory & Event, 12*(2), 1–18.

Hipsky, Martin. (2006). "Post-Cold War paranoia in *The Corrections* and *Sopranos*." *Postmodern Culture, 16*(2), 1–45.

Johnson, Merri Lisa. (2007). "Gangster feminism: The feminist cultural work of HBO's *The Sopranos*." *Feminist Studies, 33*(2), 269–296.

Killen, Andreas. (2006). *Berlin Electropolis: Shock, Nerves, and German Modernity*. Berkeley: University of California Press.

Kocela, Christopher. (2005). "Unmade men: *The Sopranos* after whiteness." *Postmodern Culture, 15*(2), 1–29.

Malkina-Pykh, I.G. and Pykh, Y.A. (2012). *The Method of Response Functions in Psychology and Sociology*. Southampton: WIT Press.

Ricci, Franco. (2014). *The Sopranos: Born under a Bad Sign*. Toronto: University of Toronto Press.

Schulman, Alex. (2010). "*The Sopranos*: An American existentialism?" *The Cambridge Quarterly, 39*(1), 23–38.

Segal, Judy Z. (2008). *Health and the Rhetoric of Medicine*. Carbondale: Southern Illinois University Press.

Strubbe, Glenn and Vanheule, Stijn. (2014). "The subject in an uproar." *Journal of the American Psychoanalysis Association, 62*(2), 237–266.

Vidler, Anthony. (1994). "Psychopathologies of modern space: Metropolitan fear from agoraphobia to estrangement." In Michael Roth (ed.), *Rediscovering History: Culture, Politics, and the Psyche*. Stanford, CA: Stanford University Press.

White, Jean. (2006). *Generation: Preoccupations and Conflicts in Contemporary Psychoanalysis*. Abingdon: Routledge.

10 *Poor Things*

Parodying diagnosis in popular culture

Hannah Tweed

In recent years the medical humanities have emerged as a rich and burgeoning field of inquiry within contemporary popular culture scholarship. As a result of the pioneering and highly influential work of theorists such as Lennard Davis (2008), Patricia Waugh (2012), and Stephen Burn (2013), cognitive disability and mental illness are increasingly recognized as crucial and recurring topics in modern and contemporary cultural productions. With the rise of *The Diagnostic and Statistical Manual of Mental Disorders* (DSM), and a diagnosis-centred culture (what T. J. Lustig and James Peacock call the "syndrome syndrome" (2013, p. 1)), an increasing number of authors are examining the stigmas surrounding hypochondria, hysteria, and medical malingering. Despite these critical trends, the diagnosis of mental illnesses and cognitive disabilities remains controversial in public discourse, and while contested illnesses are increasingly represented in literature and film, the consequences of public suspicion of these conditions are seldom explored.

Disability studies critics Sharon Snyder and David Mitchell state that "we primarily come to know disabled people, both historically and in our own moment, through representations of their lives, experiences, and bodies that have been manufactured by those outside of the immediate disability experience" (2006, p. 19). As such, one of the primary aims of disability studies is to analyse the representation and experience of disability, and to contribute to policy-making and medical treatment. Cultural disability studies aim to analyse and challenge the significance and role of representations of disability in texts and popular discourse. Drawing upon methodologies from within cultural disability studies, this chapter introduces Alasdair Gray's award-winning novel *Poor Things* (1992) as an interrogation of the complexities of modern diagnosis. While *Poor Things* has most commonly been read in terms of Scottish nationalism or postmodern aesthetics, I suggest that it also constitutes a systematic interrogation of the mutable nature of diagnostic terminology, satirizing the problems that emerge when a diagnosis becomes part of popular culture. Gray offers a parodic, anti-hierarchical critique of social norms, staged via a series of cognitively different characters, with a particular focus on hysteria and psychosomatic illnesses (and cures).

The central narrative of *Poor Things* revolves around Archibald McCandless, a nineteenth-century medical student; Godwin Baxter, a reclusive and talented surgeon; and Bella Baxter. McCandless claims that Bella is Godwin Baxter's

Frankensteinian experiment: a combination of the brain-dead body of a hysterical, neurotic, pregnant woman, recovered to technical life by Baxter, and the brain of her new-born daughter. An alternative narrative positions Bella as an amnesiac, whose mental instabilities were controversially "cured" by a head injury. *Poor Things* tracks Bella's social development and sexual education, including a period of performing as a hysteric for Charcot's private lectures. I suggest that Gray's differing representations of hysteria, hypochondria, and contested amnesia mimic and undercut common contemporary stereotypes surrounding these conditions. I also propose that Gray's postmodern, parodic illustrations – predominantly sketches of human organs, muscles, and bone – continue this examination of diagnosis and stereotypes. For example, a chapter on male hysteria is bracketed by diagrams of a penis and the medulla oblongata (the lowest section of the brain, which connects the brain to the spinal cord and controls involuntary functions such as heart rate, breathing, and blood pressure – all associated with hysteria). Through this examination of hysteria, hypochondria, and amnesia, Gray parodies the fluidity of fashionable diagnosis, and the modern drive towards medicalization.

As a novel set in Victorian Scotland, Gray is also playing with popular concepts about the nineteenth century, and particularly Victorian attitudes towards hysteria and gender. I suggest that this engagement with earlier medical practices operates as a critique of contemporary popular cultural and medical understandings of (and confusion about) psychosomatic illnesses, particularly in Western, diagnosis-centred cultures (with the rise of the DSN from the mid-twentieth century onward). Using Gray's work as an example, this chapter will demonstrate the overlap between postmodern aesthetics and the expanding sub-genre of what Stephen Burn describes as "neurologically informed fictions" (2013, p. 35), and explore the place of controversial mental illnesses and disabilities in twentieth- and twenty-first-century cultural productions.

Poor Things has been described as a classic postmodern text, despite Gray's description of postmodernism as "a specimen of intellectual afterbirth" synonymous with "fashionable" (1997, pp. 152–153).[1] Winner of the 1992 Whitbread Best Novel award and the Guardian Fiction prize, *Poor Things* received almost unreservedly positive reviews on its publication – although the reader is encouraged to question who received the praise and prizes. The prefatory note detailing the awards at the beginning of *Poor Things* also provides biographical details about "the author," one Archibald McCandless, "the illegitimate son of a prosperous tenant farmer," alongside mention of Mike Donnelly, the "Glasgow local historian" who supposedly uncovered the manuscript, the illustrator William Strang, and "the editor" Alasdair Gray (1992, p. vi).

The novel opens with the inclusion of fictitious reviews, ascribed to a mix of current, mainstream sources (*The Independent, The Scotsman*), obscure newspapers (*The Skibereen Eagle*), and clearly parodic magazines (*Private Nose, The Times Literary Implement*):

> If Gray had been content either to create a female Frankenstein or to give
> a new zest to the legend of Dr Jekyll and Mr Hyde Poor Things [*sic*] might

have been a funny and original tale. . . . But he has loaded his novel with false historical reference and larded it with his own gruesome drawings. . . . These are the ravings of second-rate characters in a second-rate novel – *Sunday Telegraph*

. . .

Fact and fiction, history and literature are stitched together and animated in that "Frankenstein method" known as post-modernism. Thus Gray remains true to his own fictional tradition, while employing the devices of older and (frankly) more accessible ones, to write this dazzling book. – *Harpers and Queens*

. . .

That intellectual hooligan, Alasdair Gray. – *The Skibereen Eagle*
(Gray, 1992, p. xv)

Such descriptors indicate to the reader that this will be a densely intertextual and self-aware novel, with a tendency to parody both realism ("false historical references") and postmodernism ("that 'Frankenstein method'") (1992, p. xv). The parodic introduction also undermines the concept of reviews as necessary statements of external approval and guides to the reader's understanding of a text. The avoidance of external judgement is compounded by the inclusion of an erratum, laid (diagonally) over the opening page of the novel, obscuring some of the reviews, and pointing out a labelling error on "page 187": 1992, p. iv). Gray's fictitious reviews reference *Frankenstein*, *Jekyll and Hyde*, and *Alice in Wonderland* – avoiding any factual touchstones, although each of the named texts does interact on some level with medical themes, albeit through fantasy. With this intertextual material, Gray satirizes a selection of cultural authority figures (editors, literary critics, medical professionals), and sets up a clear contrast to those texts that deploy specific diagnostic terminology as confirmation of authenticity and readability.

The central narrative of *Poor Things* begins with the introduction of Archibald McCandless, an impoverished medical student studying at the University of Glasgow in the late nineteenth century, and Godwin Baxter, a physically repulsive but talented surgeon, the pair of whom McCandless describes as "the two most intelligent and least social people attached to the Glasgow medical faculty" (1992, p. 11). Following an argument, the two break with each other for a number of months, before reconciling, at which point Bella Baxter (also referred to as Bella Caledonia, Bella McCandless, Victoria McCandless, Victoria Hattersley, and Lady Victoria Blessington) is introduced, and the plot becomes markedly bizarre. McCandless's text claims that Bella is the product of a spectacular and improbable experiment by Godwin Baxter: a combination of the brain-dead body of attempted suicide Victoria Blessington (née Hatterley), recovered to technical life by Baxter, and the brain of her new-born daughter, who was birthed from the dead woman's body. It does not matter whether the reader prefers that explanation of Bella's origins, or the more mundane alternative offered by her husband's lawyer and doctor (that a blow to the head rendered Bella an amnesiac, and she established a new life for herself in Glasgow, having run away from her marriage). In either scenario, in the early sections of the novel, Bella has the exuberance of a toddler in a woman's body, and a young child's idiosyncratic command of language. McCandless describes Bella's attitude and language as atypical – stating that "only idiots and infants talk like that, are capable of such radiant happiness, such frank glee and friendship on meeting someone new" (1992, p. 30). *Poor Things* tracks Bella's rapid development and her social and sexual education – which encompasses a grand European tour, an elopement, a brief stint working in a brothel, a period of performing as a hysteric for Charcot's private lectures, and her eventual return to Glasgow as the prodigal daughter, with the intention of training as a doctor. This plot trajectory conforms to some of the more socially acceptable schemes for self-enlightenment and education in the Victorian era (taking a European tour upon reaching adulthood; attending the lectures of respected and learned men) alongside the less salubrious (sexual experimentation, gambling, fiscal difficulties, and erratic letters home). With the undermining of *bildungsroman* tropes and the discretization of a range of nineteenth-century medical men – from Baxter to Charcot – Gray parodies ideas of both literary and medical authority.

The focus on medical authority in *Poor Things* is not limited to historical or literary references. The novel is filled with images that are clearly based on William Strang's paintings and engravings, complete with 'W.S.' signatures and still more fictive prefatory material crediting Strang (rather than Gray) as the artist. Gray demonstrably bases a number of his "Strang" illustrations on the actual artist's work, and still more on Henry Carter's illustrations in the first edition of Henry Gray's *Anatomy* (in the style of William Strang), and the original subjects of said engravings undercut McCandless and Gray the narrator's claims to reliability.[2] This appropriation is clearly self-aware: the most repeated image is one of a buxom woman leaning out of the mouth of a skull. The woman is presumably Bella, from the similarities to the later illustration entitled *Bella Caledonia*, and her positioning highlights the brain transplant performed by Baxter, which left Bella with the "great crack" in her skull (1992, pp. 81, 107, 220, 256. See also Appendix, figures 2 and 3). Gray, as narrator, describes this illustration as a "grotesque design" (1992, p. xvii; see also Appendix, figures 4 and 5) – a reference to the name of the Strang image on which it was based (Strang, *Grotesque*, 1897, pp. 126–127). The picture of Duncan Wedderburn is also based on a Strang engraving, entitled *Portrait of A. Jaffray*, which was painted in 1883 – the same year Gray depicts Wedderburn eloping with Bella, before Wedderburn was committed to an asylum (Strang, 1897, pp. 10–11; Gray, 1992, pp. xiv–xv, 77; see Appendix).

Gray's use of anatomical images in *Poor Things* is similarly parodic. Most of the images are inspired by (Henry) Gray's *Anatomy* (pun probably intended), and are reasonable facsimiles of sketches of human organs, muscles, and bone. Alasdair Gray's use of anatomical drawings is not merely for macabre or picaresque effect. The chapter entitled "Wedderburn's letter: Making a maniac" details Duncan Wedderburn's increasing mental instability and hysteria, and subsequent declaration of insanity. In the Preface, the narrator of *Poor Things* states of Wedderburn that 'a doctor pronounced him fit to be detained, but not to plead' (1992, pp. xiv–xv). 'Wedderburn's letter' is bracketed by a medical diagram of a penis and an image of the medulla oblongata (1992, pp. 75, 98). The medulla oblongata is the lowest section of the human brain, and connects the brain to the spinal cord, controlling involuntary functions such as heart rate, breathing, and blood pressure (OED, "Medulla oblongata,", 2013).

Typically, hysteria is characterized by "unhealthy excitement" convulsions and palpitations (OED, "Hysteria," 2013) – otherwise known as increased heart rate, hyperventilation, and a tendency to faint – and was originally conceived of as a female disease closely related to hyper-sexuality and frustrated conception. Josef Breuer, writing about severe hysteria, with additional reference to men, stated that 'in this acute stage of hysteria psychotic traits are very distinct, such as manic and angry states of excitement, rapidly changing hysterical phenomena, hallucinations, and so on' (Breuer and Freud, 1974, p. 316). Gray's illustrations suggest that Wedderburn is suffering from a male form of hysteria – only "oversexed" in this instance refers to literal exhaustion rather than to a socially unacceptable level of sexual desire, given Bella's descriptions of having "wedded" Wedderburn "until he begged [her] not to" (1992, p. 154). Similarly, the dedication of the main narration to "She who makes my life worth living" is sandwiched between detailed (and oddly beautiful) images of parts of a spleen – the "malphighian corpuscules" (1992, p. 154), to be precise.[3] Again, these images are nearly identical to Carter's anatomical drawings, but the divisive relationship between Bella/Victora (the aforementioned "She") and McCandless links as significantly to long-debunked ideas of humoral medicine as to any more modern or accurate understandings of the body.

This introduction of the spleen is particularly pertinent given classical and early modern understandings of that organ as responsible for producing "black bile," the humour associated with melancholy and hysteria (Faraone, 2011). Plato describes hysteria as the product of a "wandering womb", where that organ, "desirous of procreating children and when remaining unfruitful long beyond its proper time", becomes "discontented and angry" (1964, III: 91c). Said womb then travels "in every direction through the body, closes up the passages of the breath, and by obstructing respiration drives [women] to extremity, causing all variety of disease" (1964, III: 91c). Writing in 1733, physician George Cheyne described the spleen as one of "the more immediate and eminent causes of nervous distempers" for both men and women, prompting minor complaints such as "yawning" and a "hysterick, or nervous cough", through to more serious maladies:

[A] deep and fixed melancholy, wandering and delusory images on the brain, and instability and unsettledness in all intellectual operations, loss of memory, despondency, horror and despair, a vertigo, giddiness of staggering, vomittings of . . . choler: sometimes unaccountable fits of laughing, apparent joy, leaping and dancing; at other times, of crying, grief, and anguish; and these generally terminate in hypochondriacal or hysterical fits (I mean convulsive ones) and faintings, which leave a drowsiness, lethargy, and extreme lowness of spirits for some time afterwards.

(Cheyne, 1733, p. 183)

Cheyne's description of hysterical symptoms is markedly similar to the account of Wedderburn's behaviour at the end of his elopement with Bella. Wedderburn's rambling (and much-capitalized letter) to Baxter, having abandoned Bella in Paris, describes how Wedderburn initially alternated between "tears of gratitude" (1992, p. 87) and joy at Bella's company ('GUFFAW! GUFFAW!! GUFFAW!!!' (1992, p. 87)), and resentment of "the EXHAUSTING Bella!" (1992, p. 86). These reactions devolve into Wedderburn "sobbing" that he didn't "want to spend [his] whole honeymoon in the Midland railway terminal hotel" – forgetting, "in [his] anguish, that [they] had never married" (1992, p. 85) – before recounting a string of hallucinations and fits, for which he holds Bella responsible:

> I retreated into a corner and slowly sank to the floor, frantically punching at the space around my head as if boxing with a loathsome and swarming antagonist like huge wasps or carnivorous bats; yet I knew these vermin were not really outside but INSIDE my brain and gnawing, gnawing. . . . And Bella seemed one of them!

(Gray, 1992, p. 93)

These descriptions clearly parody the idea of hysteria as feminine weakness. Furthermore, references to discredited diagnoses, and the anatomical accuracy of Alasdair Gray's illustrations (and their similarity to Henry Gray's recognizably modern – even to a twenty-first-century reader – medical diagrams) are an ironic attempt to confirm the reliability of the narrator. Any impressions of dependability are undermined, obviously and throughout the text, by this parodying of diagnosis and the medical profession.

Poor Things also engages with the irony of discussing cognitive difference by cross-examining the concept of "normality". Bella is a perfect demonstration of the problematic definition of normal provided by the OED, as a person who is "physically and mentally sound; free from any disorder; healthy" (OED, "Normal", 2013). Few if any individuals exist in a physically ideal state. If they do, it is transitory – as highlighted by the disability rights category "Temporarily Able Bodied" (TAB), a term used with particular reference to connections between ageing and disability (Gerschick, 2000, p. 1264). Discussing the concept of the normal, Georges Canguilhem suggests that attitudes towards illness and disease have consistently reverted to the idea that "we delegate the task of restoring the diseased organism to the desired norm to technical means . . . because we expect nothing good from nature itself" (1998, p. 40). Both 'Temporarily Able Bodied' and Canguilhem's definition of normality render the totally healthy, 'normal' individual an ironic aberration. Such a description could be applied to Bella, tall and beautiful, whose 'most striking abnormality is her lack of it' (Canguilhem, 1992, p. 223). Bella, according to Baxter, has been examined by a series of medical experts, and it is the educated opinion of "Charcot of Paris, Golgi of Pavia, Kraepelin of Wurzburg, Breuer of Vienna and Korsakoff of Moscow" that Bella Baxter is "sane, strong and cheerful, with a vigorously independent attitude to life, even though amnesia (caused by injury to her skull and the loss of an unborn child) has left her with no memories preceding her arrival here" (1992, p. 222). Baxter continues his report of her mental state, declaring that these doctors had agreed that Bella:

> Shows no signs of mania, hysteria, phobia, dementia, melancholia, neurasthenia, aphasia, catatonia, algolagnia, necrophilia, coprophilia, folie de grandeur, nostalgia de la boue, lycanthropy, fetishism, Narcissism, Onanism, irrational belligerence, unhealthy reticence and is not obsessively Sapphic. They say her only obsessive trait is linguistic.
>
> (Gray, 1992, p. 222)

Such a list is ridiculous (diagnosis by default seems a distinct possibility when the medical experts offer such a plethora of labels), but, as with many of the farcical elements in *Poor Things*, it is not completely fictional – all of the listed "diagnoses" were given to patients at some point in medical history (although not, it must be granted, all at once). Furthermore, Gray's list of Bella's non-diagnoses and cross-examination of the establishment resonates with social theorist and philosopher Michel Foucault's work on the role of the medical professional in the developing legal system in nineteenth-century France. In his lectures on the "abnormal" (1974–1975), Foucault offered an analysis of the role of the expert medical witness. He argued that the role of such experts in nineteenth- and early twentieth-century France was to prove that the accused "already resembles his crime before he has committed it" (1975, p. 19). Foucault compiled the following list of quasi-diagnoses from character summaries presented to French juries by nineteenth-century psychiatrists and neurologists:

> "Psychological immaturity," "a poorly structured personality," "a poor grasp of reality." . . . "a profound affective imbalance," "serious emotional disturbance." . . . "compensation," "imaginary production," "display of perverted pride," "perverse game," "Herostratism," "Alcibiadism," "Don-Juanism," "*bovarysme*," et cetera.
>
> (Foucault, 1975, pp. 15–16)

Foucault offers this list of diagnostic terminology to demonstrate how expert witnesses used medical language as a way of proving guilt – attesting that an individual was physically and psychologically capable of committing a crime, and how that crime was in line with his or her personality. Gray's mimicry and seeming appropriation of Foucault's criticisms, parodied as they are in the form of Bella, questions medical authority, and also exemplifies a tendency in contemporary writing to parody or even pathologize the norm. Bella's improbable normality is set in direct contrast to the desire to ascribe a name to a syndrome, disability, or condition found in texts explicitly depicting disability or illness – where to be given a diagnosis, or even a specific list of symptoms or characteristics, makes one abnormal. Bella is not only strikingly normal (and therefore abnormal), but a character who is so specifically lacking a medical label that she destabilizes the concept of medical or social authority.

Furthermore, each potentially authoritative character in *Poor Things* is shown first in a position of power: Duncan Wedderburn, the lawyer in charge of writing up Baxter's will; McCandless and Baxter, both well-established medics; Bella's husband, General Blessington, with the force of law and arms behind him (and medical opinion). Yet each character fails to retain what Rosemarie Garland Thomson refers to as a "position of authority" (1997, p. 8) over Bella, and is in turn rendered not only powerless but ridiculous. Wedderburn is a failed gambler and lover who makes a hysterical fool of himself all over Europe. McCandless and Baxter are outwitted by Bella as she flees Scotland (drugging McCandless with chloroform in the process). The General, denied his wife, has his private business aired in public alongside his taste for (and embarrassment of) sado-masochism, in the guise of "Monsieur Spankybot" (1992, p. 238), and commits suicide shortly afterwards. Every instance of superior power or influence is countermanded, either by contrasting events elsewhere in the narrative, the unreliability of the narrators, or by Bella's atypical "normality". Cumulatively, this demonstrates a parodic, anti-hierarchical critique of social norms, staged via the consciousness of a cognitively different character. This constitutes a far more empowering portrayal than the more typical utilization of a specifically disabled character as a convenient foil for plot revelation or the development of a neurotypical character (both common tropes in representations of disability in popular culture (Murray, 2006)).

When Bella Baxter – the cognitively different character to trump all cognitively different characters – is diagnosed by the foremost doctors and psychiatrists of the Victorian era as "sane, strong and cheerful, with a vigorously independent attitude to life" (1992, pp. 185, 222), Gray parodies the fluidity of fashionable diagnosis and terminology. He does so not only by highlighting the irony of the premier neurologists of the Victorian era diagnosing Bella as sane (in documents "signed and witnessed with English translations attached" (1992, p. 222)), but by including a scene where Charcot – one of the aforementioned neurologists – requests that Bella "perform" neuroses for a fashionable audience. Charcot then proceeds to lecture on the hysteric symptoms of the woman he greeted as "the one completely sane English" (1992, p. 185). This parody is not simply comedic: Gray's focus on hysteria enables a cross-examination of the prioritization of diagnosis. As such, Gray engages with the potential problems that emerge when a diagnosis becomes part of popular culture, to the point where there is pressure for individuals to *perform* that diagnosis. That Bella also performs hysteria to provide Charcot with a diagnostic specimen directly references this tradition. The fact that she does so for a specious diagnosis, for profit, satirizes rather than deifies medical authority, despite the paratextual demonstration of Bella's atypical cognitive development.

This paratextual playfulness and parody is also demonstrative of Gray's engagement with postmodernism throughout *Poor Things*. Postmodernism, in potentially challenging and responding to capitalism, does so in reaction to what Linda Hutcheon refers to as the "increasing uniformisation of mass culture" (1989, p. 6). Such a process involves asserting difference, which Hutcheon describes as a "typical ... postmodern contradiction: 'difference,' unlike 'otherness,' has no exact opposite against which to define itself" (1989, p. 6). The postmodern devices featured in *Poor Things* conform to patterns of self-reflective metafictional writing, but they also serve to highlight and challenge ideas of medical authority – and the development of mass culture across the nineteenth and twentieth centuries. Such engagement is relevant to broader, contemporary representations of cognitive atypicality. The medical listing mechanisms that Gray associates with socially problematic diagnoses echo those recounted and critiqued in a range of contemporary productions, from Benjamin Kunkel's *Indecision* (2005) to the BBC series *Sherlock* (2010–2014) (among others). Cumulatively, these authors demonstrate the mutability of diagnostic terminology, and challenge the increasingly pervasive stereotypes surrounding representations of cognitive disability and illness in contemporary popular culture.[4]

Notes

1 For discussion of A. Gray as a postmodern writer, see Kaczvinsky, 2001, p. 775; and Böhnke, 2004, p. 1. For evidence of Gray's opinions on postmodernism, see Gray, 1997, p. 153, and Gray *et al.*, 2003, pp. 573–574.
2 See Appendix for details and comparative images. See also Gray, 1864, pp. 704, 718.
3 See also Gray, 1864, pp. 658–659, and Appendix, figures 6–8.
4 For further discussion of the "current preoccupation with neurological conditions and disorders" in twenty-first-century literature and film, see Lustig and Peacock, 2013, p. i. See also Kearns Miller, "Introduction," in Kearns Miller *et al.*, 2003, pp. xvii–xxiii.

References

Böhnke, D., *Shades of Gray: Science Fiction, History and the Problem of Postmodernism in the Work of Alasdair Gray* (Berlin and Wisconsin: Galda + Wilch Verlag, 2004).

Breuer, J., and S. Freud, *Studies on Hysteria*, trans. and ed. by James and Alix Strachey (London: Penguin, 1974).

Burn, S.J., "Mapping the syndrome novel", in *Diseases and Disorders in Contemporary Fiction: The Syndrome Syndrome*, ed. T.J. Lustig and James Peacock (Abingdon: Routledge, 2013), pp. 35–52.

Canguilhem, G., *The Normal and the Pathological*, trans. Carolyn R. Fawcett (New York: Zone Books, 1991, reprinted 1998).

Cheyne, G., *The English Malady: or, a treatise of nervous diseases of all kinds, as spleen, vapours, lowness of spirits, hypochondriacal, and hysterical distempers, etc.* (Cornhill: G. Strahan, 1733). Available at www.archive.org/details/englishmaladyort00cheyuoft (accessed February 28, 2015).

Davis, L., *Obsession: A History* (Chicago, IL: Chicago University Press, 2008).

Faraone, C.A., Magical and medical approaches to the wandering womb in the ancient Greek world. *Classical Antiquity*, *30*(1) (April 2011), 1–32. Available at www.jstor.org/stable/10.1525/CA.2011.30.1.1 (accessed February 28, 2015).

Foucault, M., *Abnormal: Lectures at the College de France 1974–75*, trans. Graham Burchell (London: Verso, 2003).

Garland Thomson, R*., Extraordinary Bodies: Figuring Physical Disability in American Culture and Literature* (New York: Columbia University Press, 1997).

Gerschick, T.J., "Toward a theory of disability and gender", *Signs, 25*(4) (summer 2000), 1263–1268 (p. 1264). Available at www.jstor.org/stable/3175525 (accessed February 21, 2015).

Gray, A., *Poor Things: Episodes from the Early Life of Archibald McCandless M.D., Scottish Public Health Officer* (London: Bloomsbury, 1992).

Gray, A., *Mavis Belfrage: A Romantic Novel with Five Shorter Tales* (London: Bloomsbury, 1997).

Gray, A., James Kelman, and Tom Toremans, "An interview with Alasdair Gray and James Kelman", *Contemporary Literature, 44*(4) (winter 2003), 564–586. Available atwww.jstor.org/stable/3250586 (accessed February 21, 2015).

Gray, H., *Anatomy: Descriptive and Surgical*, with drawings by H.V. Carter, 3rd edn (London: Longman, Green, Longman, Roberts, and Green, 1864).

Hutcheon, L., *A Poetics of Postmodernism: History, Theory, Fiction* (Abingdon: Routledge, 1989).

"Hysteria, n.", *OED Online* (Oxford: Oxford University Press, December 2013). Available at www.oed.com/ view/Entry/90638?redirectedFrom=hysteria (accessed February 21, 2015).

Kaczvinsky, D.P., "Making up for ;ost time': Scotland, stories, and the self in Alasdair Gray's *Poor Things. Contemporary Literature, 42*(4) (winter 2001), 775–799 (p. 775). Available at www.jstor.org/stable/1209053 (accessed February 21, 2015).

Kearns Miller, J., "Introduction", in *Women From Another Planet? Our Lives in the Universe of Autism,* ed. J. Kearns Miller *et al.* (Milan, MI: Dancing Minds Books, 2003), pp. xvii–xxiii.

Lustig, T.J., and J. Peacock, "Introduction", in *Diseases and Disorders in Contemporary Fiction,* ed. Lustig and Peacock (Abingdon: Routledge, 2013), pp. 1–16.

"Medulla Oblongata, n.", *OED Online* (Oxford: Oxford University Press, December 2013). Available at www.oed.com/view/Entry/252894?redirectedFrom=Medulla+Oblongata (accessed February 16, 2015).

Murray, S., Autism and the contemporary sentimental: Fiction and the narrative fascination of the present. *Literature and Medicine, 25*(1) (spring 2006), 24–45. Available at http://muse.jhu.edu/journals/literature_and_medicine/v025/25.1murray.html (accessed February 21, 2015).

"Normal, adj. and n.", *OED Online* (Oxford: Oxford University Press, December 2013). Available at www.oed.com/view/Entry/128269?redirectedFrom=normal (accessed February 21, 2015).

Plato, *Timaeus, Dialogues of Plato*, trans. B. Jowett (Oxford: Oxford University Press, 1964), vol. III, sect. 91c.

Snyder, S., and David Mitchell, *Cultural Locations of Disability* (Chicago, IL: Chicago University Press, 2006).

Strang, W., "Grotesque", No. 311, *William Strang: Catalogue of his Etched Work, 1882–1912* (Glasgow: James Maclehose and Sons, 1912).

Waugh, P., "Thinking in literature: Modernism and contemporary neuroscience", in *The Legacies of Modernsim: Historicising Postwar and Contemporary Fiction*, ed. David James (Cambridge: Cambridge University Press, 2012), pp. 73–95.

Appendix

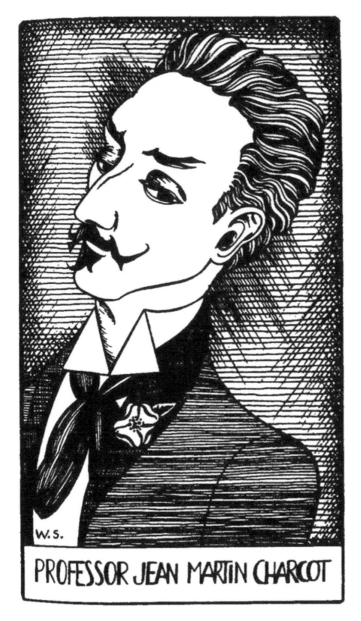

Figure 10.1 A. Gray, illustration of Robert de Montesquiou, supposedly of Jean Martin Charcot (relabelled as "Count Robert de Montesquiou-Fezensac"), *Poor Things*, p. v., 187. Based on Giovani Boldini's *Comte Robert de Montesquiou* (1987). Musée d'Orsay, "Works in Focus" series. Available at www.musee-orsay.fr/en/collections/works-in-focus/home.html (accessed 19 February 2015).

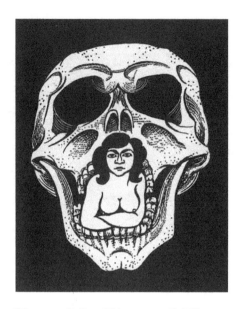

Figure 10.2 A. Gray, "Grotesque", *Poor Things,* pp. xvii, 248.

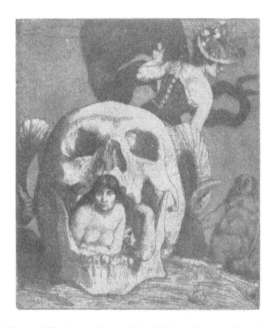

Figure 10.3 W. Strang, "Grotesque", no. 311, *William Strang: Catalogue of his Etched Work, 1882–1912* (Glasgow: James Maclehose and Sons, 1912), pp. 126–127. By permission of University of Glasgow Library, Special Collections.

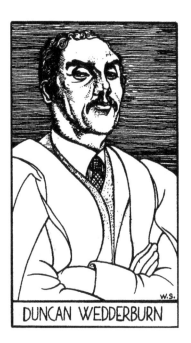

Figure 10.4 A. Gray, "Duncan Wedderburn", *Poor Things*, p. 76.

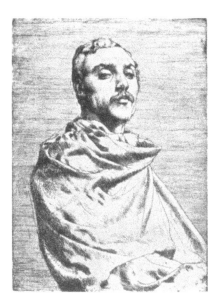

Figure 10.5 W. Strang, "Portrait of A. Jaffray", no. 25, *William Strang: Catalogue of his Etched Work*, pp. 10–11. By permission of University of Glasgow Library, Special Collections.

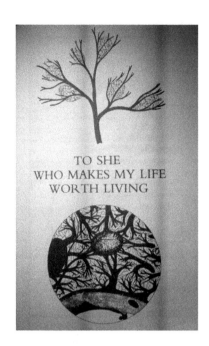

Figure 10.6 A. Gray, *Poor Things*, p. 5.

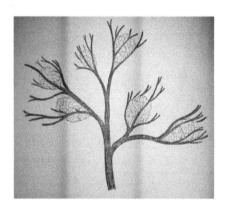

Figure 10.7 H. Gray, "348. Malpighian Corpuscles, and their Relation with the Splenic Artery and its Branches", *Anatomy: Descriptive and Surgical*, with drawings by H.V. Carter, 3rd edn (London: Longman, Green, Longman, Roberts, and Green, 1864), p. 658. By permission of University of Glasgow Library, Special Collections.

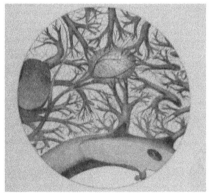

Figure 10.8 H. Gray, "349. One of the Splenic Corpuscles, showing its Relations with the Blood-vessels", *Anatomy*, drawings by H.V. Carter, p. 659. By permission of University of Glasgow Library, Special Collections.

Index

Note: page numbers in bold type refer to Figures.

physician-patient conflict 4, 5–6;
and fibromyalgia 24; and narrative
medicine 6; and patients with MSS
(multiple somatic symptoms) 12–18
physicians: education and training 14
(*see also* medicalstudentitis); frustration,
anger and burnout 17; listening skills
12; and obesity 60; television portrayals
of 76–7; *see also* narrative medicine;
primary care doctors
Plato 145–6
Poor Things (Gray) 9, 141–9, **151–4**
popular culture: and deviance 75–6;
television portrayals of physicians 76–7
Porter, D. 66
post-traumatic stress disorder (PTSD) 47,
132
postmodernism 142, 143, 148–9
postpartum depression 118
power, and diagnosis 48–9
primary care doctors: "gardening"
metaphor 52, 53; and MUS (medically
unexplained symptoms) 42, 43–4, 45,
47–8, 49–51
Propp, V. 88
psychiatry: invention of 79; and
psychosomatic illnesses 73–4, 75
psychoanalysis, and obesity 58–60
psychogenic illness 2, 3–4
Psychogenic Pain Disorder 86, 92–3, 96
psychosomatic disorder 18n1, 91–2, 94
psychosomatic illnesses 41–2;
decolonization of 71–83; definition of
128; and medical taxonomy 45–8; as
opportunity 83; performative nature of
128, 129–30, 131; and psychiatry 73–4,
75; signification in 42–3; *Sopranos,
The*/Tony Soprano case study 9,
128–38, 139–40; stigmatization
of 44
psychosomatic pain: definition 86; medical
explanations 86, 87, 92–3, 94–8;
narrative explanations 86, 87–92, 96,
98–9
psychosomatic, the 1–5, 42–3, 71, 73;
definition 66n1; stigmatization of 2, 4
PTSD (post-traumatic stress disorder) 47,
132

quest narratives 51–2

Raghinaru, Camelia 9, 128–40
Rasmussen, N. 59
Reale, Luigi 6, 23–39

realness 42–4
Rebellious Child ego state
(transactional analysis) 27–8, 30, 31
reduction, narrative 87, 95, 96, 98
Reeve, G. H. 59
reification 43, 50
repression 42
resistance to knowledge 132
rest cure 119, 122, 124
restitution narrative 9, 44, 51
rhetorical analysis 7–8
Ricci, Franco 129, 130, 137
Richardson, H. B. 59
Ricoeur, P. 86, 87, 92
rites of passage 8, 101–2; and
medicalstudentitis 104–11
Robson, Catherine 8–9, 113–27
Rubanovich, Caryn Kseniya 5–6, 12–23
Rubin, Lawrence 75–6

Sadler, J.Z. 52
Salkovskis, P. 108
Scarry, Elaine 77–8
Schick, A. 59
Schulman, Alex 136
second-year syndrome *see*
medicalstudentitis
secondary gain 94
Segal, Erich 101, 104–5, 106, 107,
109–10
Segal, Judy 128
self, the 2–3
Sepie, Amba J. 7, 71–85
shamanism 80–1, 108
Shapiro, Johanna 76
Sherlock (BBC) 149
Siberian culture 80–1
sick role 5, 50
sick-room 114–15, 124
sickness, definition 25
Simmel, Georg 138–9
sleep disturbances 132
Snelgrove, S. 94
Snyder, S.L. 5
Snyder, Sharon 141
social anxiety disorder 132
social media, patient's use of 4
Solzhenitsyn, Aleksandr 111n2
somatic metaphor 82
Somatic Symptom Disorder 18n1, 45, 47,
86, 95–6
somatic symptoms 2
somatic syndrome disorders 15
somaticization 82